LIVING LOW OXALATE

When Oxalate Rich Foods Destroy Your Health

MELINDA KEEN

The author of this book does not dispense medical advice or prescribe the use of any technique as a form of treatment for physical, emotional, or medical problems without the advice of a physician, either directly or indirectly. The intent of the author is only to offer information of a general nature to help you in your quest for emotional, physical, and spiritual well-being. A health care professional should be consulted regarding your specific situation.
ISBN: 1976596475
ISBN-13: 978-1976596476

DEDICATION

This book is dedicated to the Lord my God who held my hand, gave me strength when I had none and guided me along this path from sickness to health.

CONTENTS

ACKNOWLEDGMENTS

I want to give thanks to a loving and supportive husband, Jeff, who witnessed firsthand my journey from chronic illness to health. Thank you for encouraging me to write this message of hope and health to others who may be suffering needlessly from a little known natural food toxin called oxalate.

CHAPTER ONE

INTRODUCTION

This book was written to share how oxalates changed my life…twice, and to help others who may struggle from the effects of this toxic substance in foods you normally consider healthy. My oxalate rich diet changed me from an active, energetic, physically and emotionally healthy woman to a disabled, exhausted and chronically ill one. My life changed again when I discovered how oxalates were responsible for devastating my health. Changing my diet was the first step towards healing. If you've been diagnosed with fibromyalgia or chronic fatigue, experience bladder pain or kidney stones, or suffer with joint pain and inflammation, you should consider the possibility that it may be oxalate related. Unless you've experienced a kidney stone you may not have even heard of oxalates. Unfortunately, kidney stones are not the only health problems that people who regularly consume foods high in oxalates experience. If you're dealing with any type of inflammatory or chronic condition I encourage you to read on to discover what oxalates are, how they impact your health, and the steps necessary to walk away from their influence on chronic disease.

WHAT ARE OXALATES?

Oxalates cannot be seen, tasted, or smelled, yet people consume them almost every day. A healthy human body has the ability to manage mild levels of oxalates in foods. Some are degraded by the oxalate-degrading anaerobic bacterium that colonizes the large intestines and some are bound by minerals during digestion and are excreted. If the body isn't able to process oxalates in this manner they have a negative impact on your health. Oxalates, also called oxalic acid, are naturally occurring substances found in varying degrees primarily in plant foods such as vegetables, fruits, grains, legumes, spices, herbs, and almost all nuts and seeds. These molecules are present in the leaves, roots, stems, fruits, and seeds. Plants produce this toxic substance to provide a defense against insects and grazing animals. These needle-like crystals tear up the teeth of insects or animals which try to eat them. Most fruits and vegetables contain measurable amounts of oxalates. Some, such as rhubarb, spinach, and raspberries have especially high levels. Oxalates in foods are classified as antinutrients meaning they interfere with the absorption of vitamins, minerals, and other nutrients. They even get in the way of digestive enzymes, which are vital for proper digestion and absorption of nutrients.. There are two types of oxalates, soluble, and insoluble but the exact form of oxalate doesn't matter if one has an oxalate issue. Soluble simply means the oxalate is able to dissolve in water, and insoluble means it won't. For instance, the oxalates in tea leaves are soluble because they can be boiled out of the leaf and into the beverage. Oxalate foods lists rarely distinguish if a food consists of soluble or insoluble oxalates.

Generally, a healthy individual will not experience ill effects from small amounts of oxalates in the diet. Most people are able to safely metabolize a certain amount of oxalates in foods due to specific bacteria in the digestive tract called Oxalobacter formigenes. Problems occur when gastrointestinal microbiota has been reduced or depleted and ingested oxalates are not metabolized. Another safe way the body eliminates oxalates is the binding of it with minerals in the gastrointestinal tract. Minerals such as magnesium and calcium can bind oxalates allowing them to pass in the stool. While this inhibits absorption of these nutrients, it does insure that they are excreted rather than crossing the gastrointestinal barrier and into the blood stream. Oxalates that are not safely metabolized or bound by minerals in the gastrointestinal tract and excreted are then absorbed through the gastrointestinal barrier and enter the bloodstream. The key site for problems with accumulation of oxalates in the bloodstream is the kidneys. Blood is filtered by the kidneys where oxalates are then excreted in the urine or returned back into the bloodstream depending on the saturation level and filtration rate of the kidneys. High oxalates in the kidneys tend to combine with calcium to form calcium oxalate stones, the most common type of kidney stone. High oxalates in the bloodstream tends to bind with essential elements such as calcium, magnesium, iron, and copper and end up deposited in body tissues causing damage and exacerbating pain and inflammation. The most common location is in the joint or connective tissues, but these crystal deposits have also been found in the heart, brain, and even in the bones.[1] There are several factors that may explain why oxalates are not able to be eliminated and pass into the bloodstream.

• **Oxalate rich diet**. Oxalate rich foods are tolerated by most people as long as they are not eaten in excess or consistently over long periods of time. In excessive amounts, oxalates can build up in the blood and urine with extremely toxic results.

• **Antibiotics**. The gastrointestinal tract is home to microbes that are capable of degrading oxalates. Unfortunately, many commonly used antibiotics can kill those oxalate degrading microbes.

• **Yeast and/or fungi overgrowt**h. A lack of normal digestive bacteria, as found with chronic candida, can lead to increased oxalate availability and absorption into the blood.

• **Micronutrient deficiencies**. Dietary deficiencies of key vitamins and minerals, even small amounts, can result in unbound oxalates.

• **Fat malabsorption.** Whether due to enzyme deficiencies, pancreatic insufficiencies, liver congestion, or other diseases affecting the gastrointestinal tract, undigested fat present in the intestine will bind with calcium leaving oxalates to be absorbed into the bloodstream.

• **Leaky gut or gastrointestinal inflammation**. Oxalates can break through the delicate lining of the gastrointestinal tract if it's inflamed or injured and flood the bloodstream.

• **Prolonged constipation or diarrhea**. Digestive troubles such as constipation and diarrhea can be a sign of irritable bowel syndrome. People with irritable bowel syndrome tend to have an excessive urinary excretion of oxalate and often develop calcium oxalate kidney stones.

• **Genetics**. Primary hyperoxaluria and Dent Disease are two very rare genetic diseases that often result in life-threatening kidney stone damage. In general, these rare disorders are identified in childhood. Early diagnosis and treatment is critical.

An "oxalate-free" diet is impossible. Oxalates occur in varying amounts in almost all plant foods. If you eat food, you're almost certainly consuming oxalates in some amount. Typical diets contain upward of 200–300 mg of oxalates. A low oxalate diet usually calls for less than 50 mg of oxalates per day. This diet is usually recommended for individuals that have a history of kidney stones or increased levels of oxalic acid in their urine. Foods with the highest concentration of oxalates are also considered some of the healthiest of foods. Rhubarb, spinach, berries, nuts, chocolate, beets, and black tea have the highest amount of oxalates and are often eliminated on a low oxalate diet.

MY PERSONAL EXPERIENCE

Years ago I was suddenly struck with debilitating shoulder joint pain. I couldn't come up with any explanation for it. I could not raise my arm at all. Nothing but ice would relieve the horrible pain. Two days later, before a doctor appointment, the pain and inflammation was gone as if nothing had ever happened. Although relieved I was grateful yet still puzzled. After a few days this happened again in the other shoulder. Over and over I would experience this kind of horrible pain in various parts of my body. Sometimes it would be a finger, sometimes my whole hand, my jaw, but most often in the shoulder. There was no medical explanation. Through prayer, God led me on a journey of discovery and finally, total healing.

A year before this happened I had decided to change my mostly processed food diet to a healthier one. I took the traditional route and only ate fruits, vegetables, nuts, whole grains, and very lean meats. I practically eliminated dairy. I snacked on nuts several times a day and made sure to have spinach and sweet potatoes several times a week. I sprinkled cocoa in my morning coffee and my favorite fruits were blueberries and tangerines. Anyone who knows about oxalates would cringe at that diet.

I knew nothing about oxalates. One day I stumbled upon an article about oxalates in foods and its connection to inflammation and pain. I began to study all of the information I could find. When I found a high oxalate food list and realized my entire diet was built on these high oxalate foods, I knew I had found a connection to my disturbing health problems. I started a food and symptoms diary to be sure. At first I simply used a small notebook to record the foods I ate each day, the location of any pain, and the level of that pain using a 1-10 scale. After months of examining the food and symptoms diary I could easily see the relationship between the high oxalate foods I ate and the pain I would experience 36-48 hours later, which is the general time food is in the large intestine where remaining indigestible food matter leaves the body. I began to eliminate the foods with the highest oxalate content one week and then the medium level ones the next. Within weeks I was pain free.

I didn't expect the sudden return of that horrible pain in my right shoulder after so many weeks of living free of any pain. Perplexed, I went online to talk to others with oxalate problems and learned about the danger of going low oxalate too quickly. I was going through what is called "oxalate dumping". It was debilitating. My back began to hurt so bad I thought it was an injury so I went to see a chiropractor. The first thing he did was an x-ray. At the consultation he pulled up my x-ray, and we stood there looking at it. He seemed to be at a loss for words. I was also looking at the small white spots showing on the x-ray around my shoulders and sprinkled all over my ribs thinking about how very odd looking it was. These turned out to be calcium oxalate crystals. The source of my pain.

Calcium oxalate crystals are by far the most common factor in kidney stone formation, but my stones had formed outside of the kidneys. I learned that my steady diet of high oxalate foods had overwhelmed my system and caused my body to store the excess it could not excrete. When I stopped eating oxalate foods in the medium and high range my body had a chance to eliminate the stored oxalate crystals. It is a very painful process that can last anywhere from several days to weeks. Oxalate crystals are like tiny shards of glass. As they move they tear and inflame tissues. Since common locations of calcium oxalate stones are in joints, it's easy to assume you have osteoarthritis. Calcium oxalate is actually one of four types of crystal-associated arthritis. It's painful and debilitating. Knowing that nonsteroidal anti-inflammatory drugs (NSAIDS) were hard on the kidneys, I didn't want to use them at first. When the pain became unbearable I tried them all. Not a single one gave me relief. Later I learned that case studies report that NSAIDs seem to have very limited effectiveness on oxalate arthritis.[2]

As a nutritionist and health advocate taking a prescribed narcotic or steroid was not an option. The risk of suffering side effects and knowing they only mask the pain kept me from going in that direction. There are clearly circumstances where they are needed, but I knew I was making progress and that my body would heal with a natural approach. I sought to address the cause and focus on natural solutions. Some drug free suggestions for pain relief often recommended are turmeric, Biofreeze, arthritis creams, and Aloe vera gel. Turmeric in any amount is high oxalate and should never be taken if you have an oxalate issue. I tried Biofreeze and some arthritis creams and found very little relief. Aloe vera gel seemed to cool the inflammation down. There are many reports with reference to the anti-inflammatory effect of Aloe vera gel. In one study the gel was found to possess as effective anti-inflammatory effects as Prednisolone without having the long term toxicity of the drug.[3] I found that ice packs were the only thing that gave me dramatic pain relief. I rarely went more than three days without some level of pain, so I became rather housebound. At the worst of times, it was agonizing to get dressed, sleep, or even eat.

Excess oxalate crystals can be deposited anywhere in the body. When they do they can impair the function of whatever tissue they form in. The oddest locations of oxalate crystal pain for me were in my eye and in a saliva gland. I felt something in my eye one morning but couldn't find anything in it. After a few hours I couldn't bear it any longer, and I made my way to the nearest eye clinic. The doctor was able to remove what he said looked like a grain of sand. I'd not seen any sand since my summer vacation at the beach months earlier, so I knew it wasn't sand. My doctor was unfamiliar with calcium oxalate crystals. It had severely scratched my cornea. Months later I experienced excruciating pain near my left ear with one bite of food. After I tried a second bite a few minutes later I knew I had an emergency. I was diagnosed with a blocked salivary gland. My doctor suspected it was blocked due to a glandular infection. Treatment involved antibiotics, applying heat, drinking more fluids, and sucking on lemon drops. Two days of this was all I could stand. I took matters into my own hands and went to the mirror, applied pressure on my cheek over the swollen lump and watched the blocked duct open up. A tiny stone like a piece of glass came out. The saliva duct had been blocked by this calcium oxalate stone the same way these stones block critical parts of the kidneys.

Living low oxalate was a challenge the first year, but very successful. I continued to lower my oxalate intake until I was at the 40-50 milligrams per day or less limit, as recommended by the National Kidney Foundation to prevent kidney stone flare ups. I addressed my nutritional needs and supplemented my diet to improve the detoxification process. Gradually my health returned, and the pain has become a distant memory. Living low oxalate is a natural way of life for me now. If any of this sounds familiar to you, I strongly suggest you examine your diet for foods rich in oxalates. Since oxalates in foods have the potential to wreak havoc on your health it seems wise to use caution and limit the amount you consume. In the following pages you will find a powerful and effective health plan that addresses oxalate issues in the body.

CHAPTER TWO

SYSTEMIC DISTURBANCES

No benefit has been found for oxalates in the body. In fact, they disrupt normal bodily functions on the cellular level affecting health on a broader, systemic level. Systemic disturbances occur when oxalates are absorbed into the bloodstream via the gastrointestinal tract. If gastrointestinal bacteria has been compromised either by alcohol consumption, yeast overgrowth, poor diet, or antibiotic use, oxalates will not be degraded. The body will respond with protective measures such as binding the oxalate with minerals. Calcium, iron, and magnesium are the most common minerals that bind with oxalates. These bonds of oxalate and minerals in the gastrointestinal tract are then excreted in the stool. Unbound oxalates have the potential to pass through the gastrointestinal barrier and enter the bloodstream causing numerous problems.

Over consuming high oxalate foods for an extended period of time can also overwhelm the body's ability to degrade or eliminate them. This results in increased levels of oxalates in the blood, urine, and in bodily tissues. Some people are unaware of oxalate accumulation until they have reached their own tipping point and symptoms arise. These powerful and very reactive molecules can wreak havoc on your health.

Varied effects of high oxalates in cells and tissues:

- Interferes with and damages mitochondrial function, thereby impairing cellular energy
- Creates oxidative stress
- Results in digestive issues
- Disrupts mineral absorption and usage
- Depletes nutrients like glutathione and the B vitamins
- Damages tissues
- Causes histamine release

Clinical studies indicate that mitochondrial disruption and damage, oxidative stress, and nutrient depletions trigger widely varied symptoms, including fatigue and inflammatory cascades, joint pain, or pain anywhere in the body. Mitochondria are compartments within almost every cell of the human body. They are often called the powerhouse of cells because they help with the process of creating energy within cells. Once oxalate gets into cells where it can disrupt mitochondrial function; it can cause all sorts of systemic disturbances.[4] Chronic low energy is a very common result of a diet high in oxalate rich foods because of its ability to reduce ATP (intracellular energy) in the mitochondria.

Oxalates generate free radicals. Free radicals are like waste products from various chemical reactions in the cell. When free radicals increase the burden your body experiences is called oxidative stress. Oxidative stress harms the cells and is associated with diseases such as autoimmune conditions and inflammatory bowel disorders such as ulcerative colitis and Crohn's disease. These conditions are characterized by inflammation of the lining of your digestive tract. Leaky gut is a common term for the condition of the small intestine where the intestinal tract has been damaged and thus allows larger than usual food molecules and toxins to enter the blood stream. The causes of these digestive diseases and conditions are unknown but linked to urinary tract stones. Based on the reports of clinical trials, calcium oxalate is more prevalent in Crohn's Disease.[6] Oxalate crystals can be razor sharp and may be the cause of damage to the gastrointestinal tract. An inflamed or permeable intestinal lining will allow these crystals to pass through, enter the bloodstream and form stones in the renal system. The National Institutes of Health estimates that nearly ¼ of us (about 70 million) suffer from digestive issues: gas, bloating, heartburn, diarrhea, constipation, and nausea.[5] A cluster of these symptoms is commonly labeled Irritable Bowel Syndrome. Gastrointestinal imbalances have been linked to hormonal imbalances, autoimmune diseases, diabetes, chronic fatigue, fibromyalgia, abdominal pain, anxiety, and depression just to name a few. Individuals as well as practitioners should examine oxalate influence as the potential source of such common symptoms due to their toxicity and inflammatory influence.

If you suffer from autoimmune conditions or inflammatory bowel disorders a trial on a low oxalate diet may put you on the right tract to healing. Withdrawing from oxalate rich foods, even for as short as two weeks, can determine whether oxalate influence is at the root of your problem. If you eliminate oxalate rich foods and feel better, the next step would be to heal your gastrointestinal tract.

A properly functioning digestive system is critical to good health. The vast bulk of mineral absorption occurs in the small intestine. Specific vitamins work in synergy with minerals. The presence of oxalates in the small intestine disrupts this synergy by binding with minerals. Oxalates bind with calcium and magnesium, as well as iron and copper preventing them from being absorbed properly in the intestinal tract. This can lead to mineral deficiencies, such as calcium and/or magnesium deficiency. Oxalates also change how zinc works within the body, which can affect immune function.

Oxalates also deplete glutathione, an antioxidant, and B vitamins. Glutathione is the key antioxidant in the detoxification process. The body's toxicity increases as glutathione and B vitamins are depleted. Vitamin B6, vitamin B12, and folate are important for maintaining glutathione levels. Toxicity affects the immune system. A weakened, worn out, overloaded immune system is slow to respond to a toxic invasion or will not respond at all. If the immune system is compromised, the body's second line of defense is stimulated into action and inflammation sets in. Internal cell damage begins often resulting in tissue destruction and diseases. More and more disease states point to excessive oxalates, and more and more doctors are asking if this condition could be from high oxalates.[7]

When the blood delivers oxalate crystals to bodily tissues damage results due to the sharp slivers of glass structure. When kidney stones pass from the kidney, they cause pressure and pain in the bladder and urethra and can actually tear up the walls of the urinary tract. Oxalate crystals which end up in the thyroid can cause thyroid disease by damaging thyroid tissue. Affected areas are more common in the urinary system but oxalates have also been found in bones, joints, tendons, heart, eyes, and skin.

Oxalates entering the blood from the gastrointestinal tract will cause the immune system to releases histamine. It's a natural reaction to these foreign bodies. Histamines are chemicals produced by the body during an allergic reaction, generally causing itchiness, redness, swelling, rash, and cough in response to various allergens. These reactions are part of the inflammatory response. Histamines travel throughout the bloodstream and therefore can affect the gastrointestinal tract, lungs, skin, brain and entire cardiovascular system. Histamine often manifests in a wide array of health problems with vague symptoms such as migraines, constipation, diarrhea, nausea, and skin rashes that are difficult to diagnose. Oxalates can be a hidden source of headaches, urinary pain, genital irritation, and joint, muscle, intestinal, or eye pain.

Other common oxalate-caused symptoms may include mood conditions, anxiety, sleep problems, weakness, or burning feet. Many of the problems caused by oxalates go misdiagnosed because they are easily associated with aging. It's also easy to assume that certain problems are the result of better known causes that create similar symptoms. If you are not finding relief through your doctor it's quite possible your condition is oxalate related. The best way to find out if you are affected by oxalates is to slowly change to a low oxalate diet. If your symptoms improve you will be on the right path to wellness.

CHAPTER THREE

THE OXALATE INFLUENCE ON CHRONIC DISEASE

Oxalates can be a contributing factor to kidney stones, bladder irritation and pain, joint pain, chronic fatigue, fibromyalgia, gastrointestinal distress, autism and other developmental disorders, and much more. Having a greater understanding of their influence may pave the way to your own awareness that oxalates lie at the root of your illness. If you find your symptoms improving by lowering your oxalate intake you may have found the roadblock to your health.

CALCIUM OXALATE KIDNEY STONES

The four types of kidney stones are uric acid stones, struvite stones, cystine stones and calcium oxalate stones. Stones can be analyzed giving your doctor the information needed for treatment. Management of stone disease should be handled by a physician. The information in this book only addresses the calcium oxalate kidney stone. Calcium oxalate kidney stones are the most common type of kidney stone. About 80% of kidney stones are partially or entirely of the calcium oxalate type. This type of kidney stone is formed when oxalate binds to calcium while urine is produced by the kidneys. When undigested or unbound oxalates enter the bloodstream they travel to the kidneys to be removed as waste in the urine. If there is an abundance of oxalate and calcium in the urine, these will bind together to form a solid mass. Changing your diet can prevent the recurrence of this type of stone.

Unless you've had a kidney stone, you probably haven't spent a lot of time wondering about what causes them, what they're made of or how to prevent them. There are many potential causes of kidney stone formation. Hyperoxaluria, too much oxalate in your urine, can be caused by an intestinal disease, eating too many oxalate-rich foods, or an inherited genetic disorder. Quick diagnosis and treatment is important to the long-term health of your kidneys. Treatment for hyperoxaluria that's caused by intestinal disease or eating too many oxalate-rich foods usually includes following a low oxalate diet.[8] Primary hyperoxaluria, or oxalosis, is a rare genetic disorder found mainly in children. The kidneys of these children fill with stones due to the body generating too much oxalate. Identifying and treating any underlying disease would be the first step in correcting a kidney abnormality.

BLADDER IRRITATION AND PAIN

Interstitial cystitis, also called painful bladder syndrome, is a chronic irritation of the bladder that causes urinary frequency, urgency, pressure, and pain. Sometimes pelvic pain and inflammation is involved as well. The bladder pain can range from mild discomfort to severe. When urine is normal and infection is not the main cause, some researchers have suggested that it may be related to the endocrine factors, autoimmune disease, or cancer. Therefore, it should be emphasized that a biopsy of cells from inside the bladder should be done.

Research indicates that oxalates can form throughout the kidneys, in the urinary tract, and in the bladder as well. These star-shaped crystalline stones can be the cause of pain and pressure in the urinary tract. They are known to tear into the walls of the urinary tract itself, and end up in the bladder where they are likely to cause the symptoms of interstitial cystitis. Diuretic and Anti-inflammatory medications are the typical treatments for patients who are suffering from interstitial cystitis. Following a low-oxalate diet may determine if oxalates are the source of interstitial cystitis. If symptoms improve, this may be the only treatment necessary.

The presence of calcium oxalate crystals in urine has been linked to an oxalate-rich diet.[9] A load of oxalates can be excreted in the urine occasionally but over time, excessive urinary oxalate can damage the kidneys, urinary tract, and the bladder due to the extremely sharp structure. Severe pain and inflammation is a result of oxalate crystals moving against or embedding in body tissues. A diet low in oxalates has been suggested for bladder pain and as a treatment for women who experience unexplained vulval pain or vulvodynia.[10]

JOINT PAIN AND INFLAMMATION

Calcium oxalate crystal deposits can occur within a variety of body tissues. Oxalates are primarily eliminated in the gastrointestinal tract and in the stool, but when this doesn't happen oxalates enter the bloodstream potentially accumulating anywhere in the body.

Calcium oxalate crystal arthritis can result from deposit of calcium oxalate crystals within bones, tendons, cartilage or the fluid in the joints of the shoulder, elbow, wrist, knee, or ankle. A deposit in a tendon can cause it to bulge and become inflamed. An inflamed tendon between bones make it difficult and painful to move. Calcium oxalate crystal arthritis sometimes called pseudo-gout, may be more painful and severe than most osteoarthritis.[11] It can be diagnosed by synovial fluid, lubricating fluid secreted by membranes in joint cavities, analysis. The best treatment for increased absorption of dietary oxalate is a low oxalate diet. An intake of foods very high in oxalates can result in a substantial oxalate load. This was my own experience. The crystals are thought to gain entry into the fluid of joints where they invoke an inflammatory response. Super saturation of calcium oxalate within synovial fluid itself may lead to local crystal formation or calcification around the joints, within tendon sheaths, and in soft tissue. Calcium oxalate crystals have been found in the spine, along the ribs, and even inside bones.[12]

Other issues caused by calcium oxalate crystals being deposited elsewhere in the body are a rare metabolic disorder called oxalosis and renal failure. Because the kidneys stop functioning correctly, the blood calcium oxalate supersaturation level exceeds the point of normal fecal and urine elimination, and the body begins to deposit these stones elsewhere.[13]

CHRONIC FATIGUE

Chronic fatigue syndrome is a debilitating disorder characterized by extreme fatigue or tiredness that doesn't go away with rest and can't be explained by an underlying medical condition. Other symptoms of chronic fatigue may include muscle pain, frequent headaches, multi-joint pain, frequent sore throat, and swollen lymph nodes in the neck and armpits. Potential causes of chronic fatigue are a key part of the diagnosis process. Some conditions whose symptoms resemble those of chronic fatigue include mononucleosis, Lyme disease, lupus, and fibromyalgia. Each afflicted person may benefit from different types of treatment aimed at managing the disease and relieving their symptoms. There is currently no specific cure for chronic fatigue and no medication has successfully treated this illness. Inflammatory cascades, joint pain, and pain in various parts of the body are symptoms often relieved by anti-inflammatory drugs, anticonvulsants, antidepressants, and narcotics.

Clinical studies indicate that oxidative stress, mitochondrial disruption and damage, and nutrient depletions trigger widely varied symptoms including chronic fatigue. Chronic low energy is very common in mitrochondrial dysfunction. If you suffer from chronic fatigue or have been diagnosed with this syndrome it may be beneficial to understand and consider the influence of oxalates in cellular energy.

Once oxalates get into cells they can disrupt mitochondrial function, produce inflammation, and can impair cellular energy. Oxalates in cells impairs cellular energy by depleting nutrients like the antioxidant, glutathione. Glutathione deficiency leads to increased oxidative stress and a greatly reduced ability to detoxify the body. When cellular energy is impaired there is a reduced supply of oxygen and nutrients available to the cells. The result of impaired cellular energy and oxidative stress is commonly called chronic fatigue. The immune system will also trigger an inflammatory response to oxalates inside cells which results in swelling, redness, aches and pains. An accumulation of oxalate crystals in the muscle and connective tissue cells may be the cause of the muscle aches and pain associated with Fibromyalgia.

FIBROMYALGIA

Fibromyalgia, also called fibromyalgia syndrome (FMS), is a long-term condition that causes chronic pain all over the body. Associated symptoms of FMS include chronic fatigue, headaches/migraines, brain fog, yeast overgrowth, insomnia, and hormone imbalance. It can be a debilitating condition, involving many systems within the body. The pain can be every bit as bad as arthritis yet doesn't seem to have a physiological cause. It's not clear exactly how many people are affected by fibromyalgia, although research has suggested it could be a fairly common condition. Some estimates suggest nearly 1 in 20 people may be affected by fibromyalgia to some degree. Fibromyalgia can be a difficult condition to diagnose, making it unclear as to just how many people are affected by it. It's also very resistant to treatment. Treatment tends to be a combination of pain medications and exercise. Many who have struggled with the pain of fibromyalgia have actually found relief when adopting a low-oxalate diet.[14] If oxalate crystals are deposited in muscle tissue normal movement would cause inflammation and exercise would be very painful. Dr. Clare E. Morrison, a general practitioner from the UK who has fibromyalgia, found relief from symptoms after changing to a low-oxalate diet. She tells her story of self diagnosis and recovery online in a 2012 article in the health section of Daily Mail. The body can, over time, detoxify itself of oxalates with a combined low oxalate diet and supplementing with the right nutrients. High oxalate levels in the body can be a factor in many chronic conditions. Accumulation of oxalates in bodily tissues can interfere with cellular functions affecting health on such a broad level.

AN AUTISM CONNECTION

Although the metabolic pathways are unclear, individuals with autistic tendencies have seen an improvement in their symptoms when consuming a low oxalate diet. Up to 84% of those on the autism spectrum concurrently have elevated oxalate levels. These kids do not necessarily have the genetic condition called Primary Hyperoxaluria but do tend to have very high levels of oxalate that can aggravate or cause autism-like symptoms. Most of the autism and oxalate research has been done by a researcher named Susan Owens. She discovered that many ASD children significantly improved with a low oxalate diet.

Researcher Susan Owens discovered that the use of a diet low in oxalates markedly reduced symptoms in children with autism. Some of the benefits reported by parents using the low oxalate diet were improvements in sleep, counting ability, expressive speech, and fine motor skills.

CHAPTER FOUR

LOWERING YOUR OXALATE INTAKE

After examining a few oxalate content food lists, many of you may be thinking you will never be able to eat fruits or vegetables again. The truth is almost everything, high oxalate or not, can be incorporated into your diet safely. The highest oxalate foods such as spinach, beets, rhubarb, chocolate, especially dark chocolate, and most nuts are the only ones that must be eliminated. Chocolate and nuts are the hardest for most people to give up. These alone often discourage one from even trying a low oxalate diet. It's going to take motivation to change and stay with a low oxalate way of eating. To me, pain was the great motivator. As much as I love chocolate and never imagined a day without it, I no longer give it a thought. Once when I thought I was finally free from oxalate pain, I ate one of those mini chocolate bars. It didn't take long to realize I'd made a terrible mistake. After that experience, I was determined to stay away from chocolate, even white chocolate, fearing similar results. However, white chocolate isn't the same. It's made with cocoa butter and milk, and sweetened with sugar and vanilla which makes it oxalate free. Cocoa powder is the ingredient in chocolate that's rich in oxalates. There are other swaps that you can make (see chapter 7) from higher to lower oxalate foods. The goal you want to achieve is to lower your oxalate consumption to 40-50 mg or less each day.[15] Most of your food choices will come from the low and medium oxalate food categories. You may also choose some foods in the high and even very high oxalate foods category as long as the daily oxalate intake does not exceed 50 mg. Watching portion sizes and keeping track of the total amount of oxalates consumed daily is necessary.

You don't have to be a master chef in order to live a low oxalate life, but you will likely have to learn how to prepare most of your own food. Almost every processed food is high in oxalates or has oxalate containing foods listed in the ingredients. Once you're familiar with the oxalate content of foods and get past the ups and downs of recovery, you will find living low oxalate easy. Read food labels when choosing processed foods and watch for the very high oxalate foods, such as soybeans, brown rice flour, nuts or nut flours, and cinnamon. Eating out can be a challenge. Finding green bell pepper in your guacamole, spinach in your soup, or sesame seeds on your bun will be disheartening. You'll have to decide on whether to eat it or order something else. Asking about ingredients before ordering or ordering something you are sure is low oxalate is the only way to eat out safely.

The first steps on your low oxalate journey towards health must be small. Slowly, as in weeks rather than days, step down your oxalate intake. Start with one or two high oxalate foods you have been eating and eliminate them. The oxalate contents of foods lists (chapter 6) will help. After a week or two, start swapping out higher oxalate foods for lower ones. You may not have your overall oxalate intake under 50 mg yet that's all right. Continue lowering your intake a little more each week or two until you average 40-50 mg each day. You may begin to feel better right away, but soon your body will see this as an opportunity to get rid of any stored oxalates. When oxalate crystals begin to break apart, move out of storage and into your bloodstream, and towards excretion, you may experience a worsening of symptoms. This has been referred to as "dumping" or "crystal shedding". Reducing oxalate levels too quickly can cause the body to dump too much at once and cause severe issues such as pain, inflammation, and possibly kidney stones. Your kidneys can only filter so much at one time. Give your body time to adjust to each change. The body will gradually break down and remove these toxic crystals. Depending on how fast you can detoxify and how much oxalate you have stored, it could take a few months to possibly a year or more to get your health back. You can expect to go through times of great relief followed by short returns of previous symptoms. The period of relief will grow longer each time until all oxalate stores have been removed and health has been restored. Sometimes relief of symptoms is quick and long-lasting making it easy to forget to continue eating low oxalate. Even though it may be a bit time consuming, I suggest you keep a food and symptoms diary. Daily record the foods you eat, the oxalate content of each, and record your symptoms or pain level. This will help you stay focused and allow you to associate symptoms with certain foods. I used a small spiral bound notebook. On the pages to the right, I recorded the day of the week and simply listed the foods I consumed on that day. If the food had an oxalate value between 2-12 mg (medium-high range) I made a note so as not to exceed the 40–50 mg of oxalate per day recommendation. On the pages to the left, I recorded any symptoms I had that day no matter what they were. When there was pain I rated it on a scale of 1-10 and looked back to examine which food may have caused it. If you feel the temptation to abandon the low oxalate diet, take out your food and symptoms diary to remind yourself how far you've come.

Cooking methods can change oxalate levels in different ways. Frying, baking, microwaving, or soaking will not destroy the oxalates, or alter the amount of oxalates present but boiling and sometimes steaming can. Boiling markedly reduces the soluble oxalate content of some food by 30−87% and is more effective than steaming (5−53%).[16] It's very important to discard the boiling water if you use this method. Not knowing the exact oxalate content of the boiled food is the only drawback. When boiling a food, the serving size may be different than what it's listed as on an oxalate food value list. A condensed product, such as a cup of boiled leafy greens would have a higher oxalate content than a cup of raw leafy greens. So even though boiling will reduce the oxalates of greens, you would also need to reduce the serving size as well. Again, the amount of oxalate cannot be accurately determined with this method. I was delighted to add potato salad back into my diet because boiling it reduces the oxalate content yet does not condense it. Even though it's popular to roast certain vegetables, keep in mind that the total oxalate levels of vegetables such as Brussels sprouts, broccoli and carrots can be reduced by boiling. Another thing to consider is that jams, jellies, and sunbutter are condensed forms of the food making them higher in oxalates than in the original state.

Never ignore your body's signals. If familiar oxalate symptoms arise, your body may be telling you that something you are eating is high in oxalates. Despite how some foods are listed in a list, I highly recommend going with your own judgment. All foods are products of their own makeup, as well as the soil in which they were grown. This means that a white onion grown in Texas may have a different level of oxalates than one grown in Idaho. This is one of the many reasons I advise keeping a food and symptoms diary. Once you begin paying attention to the signals your body sends, you may just be surprised at how much more you can learn. I found that cranberry sauce produced pain and inflammation even though cranberries are listed as low oxalate. With a food and symptoms diary it's easy to look back 36-48 hours from a symptom to see which food might have caused the issue. The average transit time from ingestion to the large intestine, or colon, where oxalates have the potential to pass into the bloodstream to circulate freely, is 33-47 hours. Oxalates leaving the gastrointestinal tract then quickly bind to minerals, reach the bladder, or lodge in bodily tissues causing immediate inflammatory conditions.

CHAPTER FIVE

THE JOURNEY TO WELLNESS

In addition to using the following oxalate content of foods lists to gradually lower your oxalate intake to less than 50 mg of oxalate per day, there are several things that should be addressed to improve health. Exercise and proper nutrition, along with lowering your toxic burden, will support your journey to wellness and optimize the processing of any stored oxalates in the body.

EXERCISE AND NUTRITION

Common health advice such as exercise and proper nutrition are vitally important. According to an analysis of a large cohort study, physically active women had about a 30% lower risk of kidney stones compared with women who reported no exercise. The risk reduction ranged as high as 80% in one analysis, reported Mathew Sorensen, MD, of the University of Washington in Seattle and colleagues at the American Urological Association meeting.[17] If you want to exercise every day, go for it, but make sure to listen to your body. Any amount of pain should be heeded as a warning to stop. Calcium oxalate crystal deposits are very abrasive. They can degrade a joint if you continue to exercise when pain is present. Walking is the gentlest form of exercise. It improves fitness, cardiac health, alleviates depression and fatigue, creates less stress on joints, and reduces pain. Yoga exercises have become popular lately due to the benefits of improved strength, flexibility, and balance. Flowing from one pose to the next at your own pace is a great way to increase blood flow, increase the drainage of lymph and aid in digestive health. A yoga mat, rug or thick carpeting, some space, and a good instruction book or video is all that's needed to practice at home. Regular practice of yoga exercise can also maintain or improve antioxidant levels in the body.[18]

Moderate physical exercise, without increased fluid intake to compensate for excessive sweating, may cause the crystallization of calcium oxalates in urine so be sure to drink plenty water. Drinking plenty of water and limiting sodium in your diet will thin out your urine and make it harder for any more oxalates to build up and form crystals.[19]

The foundation of a healthy diet is real food nutrition. Real food is simple, unprocessed, whole food that is nutrient rich, low in sugar, high in fiber, and loaded with antioxidants. Replacing processed food with real food, preferably organic, whenever possible makes a huge impact on health. Herbicides and pesticides used on crops remain on fruits and vegetables even after they are washed. USDA resources found a total of 178 different pesticides and pesticide breakdown products on the thousands of produce samples they had analyzed.[20] There is no legal limit on the number of different pesticides allowed on food. The effects of these chemicals are unknown, but eating organic is one of the best ways to lower your overall toxic burden because synthetic chemicals are not allowed on organic foods. Pesticide exposure has been linked to nerve damage and some cancers.[21] Conventionally raised meats are often given drugs and hormones to grow faster, as well as antibiotics. Their diets are based on corn and soy, usually treated with pesticides, which are not the animal's natural diet. In the U.S., the majority of both corn and soy are genetically modified.[22] Organic meats and eggs reduce your exposure to hormones, antibiotics, and pesticides. Growth hormones and antibiotics are prohibited under organic regulations. Grass-fed cows, wild-caught fish, and pasture-raised poultry eat a natural diet free of pesticides and genetic modification. Lessening this toxic burden gives the body a chance to detoxify and reset health. Our bodies constantly require nutrients to function and must be supplied with wholesome food for optimal performance and health. Supplying your body with good nutrition gives your body the building materials to restore health.

There are 6 basic nutrients required for good health.

Water
Carbohydrates
Proteins
Fats
Vitamins
Minerals

When you reduce the amount of oxalates in your diet, you are reducing a totally non-nutritive substance that contributes directly to health issues. Replacing oxalate rich foods with nutrient dense foods will help nourish your body and restore your health. The greater the variety in your diet, the better chance you have of getting all your necessary nutrients.

Water

Water is essential to your health. Approximately 60 percent of the body is made of water. It maintains the body's fluid balance, which helps transport nutrients in the body, regulate body temperature, digest food, and more. It's even more important to drink plenty if you suffer oxalate related illness. The National Kidney Foundation recommends drinking at least 10-12 cups of water daily can help dilute any oxalates in the blood and flush it out of your body. This will also reduce your risk of forming kidney stones. The kidneys process about 200 quarts of blood daily, sifting out waste and transporting urine to the bladder. Therefore the kidneys need plenty of fluids to clear away what we don't need in the body. Citric acid in lemon is known to help prevent the formation of calcium oxalate stones so adding fresh squeezed lemon juice to your water would be an added benefit.[23]

Carbohydrates

Carbohydrates provide the body with energy and are a good source of many vitamins and minerals. They are considered the body's most preferred source of energy for all metabolic functions. Approximately 50% of the energy obtained by the foods we eat are derived from carbohydrates and the remaining 50% is derived from proteins and fats. Choose vegetables and fruits over whole grains which tend to be high in oxalates. Good sources of carbohydrates are bananas, peas, lentils, white rice, and pasta as long as it's not whole grain pasta. Rice pasta and egg noodles are low oxalate alternatives to whole grain pasta. Dietary fiber is a type of carbohydrate that the body can't digest. It adds bulk to your diet, makes you feel full faster, helps digestion, and helps prevent constipation. Getting an adequate amount of fiber can be a challenge on a diet that restricts oxalate, as many fiber-rich foods also happen to be high in oxalate. Pears, apples, red bell peppers, and asparagus are high in fiber and low in oxalates.

Protein

Protein is important for repair, maintenance, and growth of cells and is essential for healthy muscles, organs, glands, and skin. Consuming a moderate amount of protein by eating beef, fish and poultry, milk, cheese, and eggs can provide high-quality protein. Plant based foods high in protein as well as fiber include lima beans, pumpkin seeds, broccoli, avocados, and Brussels sprouts.

Fats

Eating healthy, high-quality fat is crucial. Inflammatory omega-6 fats in vegetable oils such as canola and soybean oils should be eliminated and replaced with anti-inflammatory oils such as olive and coconut oil. Extra virgin olive oil is loaded with antioxidants, some of which have powerful health benefits. Omega-3 fats found in salmon and other wild-caught, cold-water fish as well as grass-fed beef and dairy have been shown to reduce muscle, bone, and joint pain by lowering inflammation.[24] Studies show that a lower ratio of omega-6s to omega-3s can reduce the risk of many chronic diseases. A team of researchers at Bonn University in Germany report that supplementing with omega 3 rich fish oil can reduce the risk of supersaturation of calcium oxalate in the urine by as much as 14%, thus reducing the risk of kidney stones.[25]

Vitamins

Oxalates cause the body to lose vitamin B6, which among other functions is essential for energy production. Low levels of vitamin B6 have been associated with increased symptoms of rheumatoid arthritis, including more severe pain. If supplementing with B6, which I don't advise, the current recommended maximum daily intake is 100 mg. High doses of the B6 vitamin can, over time, become toxic and may result in nerve damage. There is no evidence of any adverse effect from consuming too much vitamin B6 in food. Foods rich in B6 are bananas, milk, cheese, eggs, chicken, turkey, grass-fed beef, avocado, and salmon. The only vitamin supplement I would recommend is vitamin K2 as MK-7 (menaquinone-7). Vitamin K2 is critical for balancing out the effects of vitamin D and making sure the calcium from our diet gets deposited into our bones and not into our arteries. Vitamin K2 goes straight to the vessel walls, bones, and tissues other than the liver. It has been shown to remove calcifications like bone spurs and kidney stones. The MK7 form of vitamin K2 also prevents inflammation.[26] There is no actual recommended daily allowance (RDA) for vitamin K2. If you take a vitamin K2 supplement I strongly recommend increasing your intake of calcium rich foods to achieve balanced nutrient levels. If you are on blood thinning medication you should speak to your doctor before taking a vitamin K supplement as this can change the effects of the medication. The best way to increase your vitamin K2 is to consume grass-fed dairy products like ghee, butter, and full-fat cheeses as well as fermented foods such as kimchi and sauerkraut.

Vitamin C is vital for health. It helps form and maintain bones, skin, and blood vessels. It synthesizes collagen, metabolizes protein and improves iron absorption. Viamin C is also an important antioxidant that promotes overall health and may also be beneficial in supporting healthy immune function. Vitamin C is a water-soluble vitamin that isn't stored by the body and must continually be replaced. The Recommended Daily Allowance (RDA) for vitamin C in adults is 90 mg/day for men and 75/mg day for women. Foods high in vitamin C and low in oxalates include red or yellow bell peppers, cauliflower, cabbages, Brussels sprouts, pineapple, lemon, cantaloupe, and watermelon. Getting your vitamin C from foods instead of a supplement is very important if you have issues with oxalates. Dietary vitamin C intake has not been associated with kidney stone risk but supplements have been known to raise the amounts of oxalate in the urine.[27] It's critically important to abstain from vitamin C supplements.

Minerals

Because oxalates bind to minerals, especially calcium and magnesium, you may have a deficiency. The ability of these minerals to bind to oxalates in the gastrointestinal tract leaves less available for absorption. Simultaneous ingestion of calcium rich foods with meals is important. Eating calcium rich foods such as dairy products, broccoli, and low oxalate leafy greens like romaine and bok choy, will easily bind oxalates in a meal. The calcium oxalate stones formed in the upper intestine will then safely pass in the stool. It may seem easier to increase your calcium by taking a supplement. However, calcium in the form of a supplement may raise your chances of forming new calcium oxalate stones.[28] Some people take calcium citrate supplements with a meal to bind with the oxalates, but this comes with many risks. Possible side effects include upset stomach, constipation, increased urination, and unusual tiredness. Calcium from food sources have positive effects and are best because you get the added nutrients as well. The adult recommended dietary allowance (RDA) for calcium is 1,000–1,200 mg per day. Three servings of dairy daily would add 900 milligrams of calcium to your diet. Other low oxalate foods that can help you meet your daily requirement for calcium are canned salmon, black eyed peas, and blackstrap molasses. Since calcium citrate is the calcium salt derived from citric acid, foods rich in naturally-occurring citric acid contain calcium citrate. These include lemons, limes, and grapefruit. Lemon juice contains 1.44 grams per ounce of calcium citrate. I highly recommend squeezing the juice of one lemon in a glass of water with a meal. The calcium citrate will help bind with any oxalate and supply you with approximately 13 mg of vitamin C as well.

Magnesium is extremely important for health, and especially so on a low oxalate diet. The recommended daily requirement for magnesium is approximately 400 mg per day for men and 300 mg per day for women. This is basically a minimum recommendation. Magnesium levels in the body are depleted by antibiotics, painkillers, stress, sugar, and highly processed foods. Low magnesium levels are believed to impair the ability to absorb and use vitamin B6. Magnesium is essential for over 300 biochemical functions in the body.

Some of the major functions that require magnesium are:

- Nerve function
- Neurotransmitter release
- Blood pressure regulation
- Energy metabolism
- Production of the antioxidant glutathione

Supplementing with magnesium is even more crucial when you start lowering oxalate intake because many magnesium rich foods are also high in oxalates. Spinach, almonds, and chocolate are some of the richest food sources of magnesium, but these same foods are also high in oxalates. Magnesium rich and low oxalate food sources of magnesium include avocado, pumpkin seeds, bok choy, salmon, romaine, Brussels sprouts, and broccoli.

Another important factor for supplementing with magnesium is that it is an inhibitor of calcium crystal growth.[29] In the book *The*

Magnesium Miracle, Dr. Carolyn Dean M.D. N.D, a medical and naturopathic doctor, discusses the importance of this mineral and how it also breaks down stored oxalate crystals by making them more soluble. It's a mineral with very low toxicity as long as an individual's kidneys are functioning properly. Excess magnesium that the body cannot use is generally excreted in the urine or stool.

There are at least 9 common types of magnesium supplement. Magnesium in its elemental form isn't stable by itself. It has to be bound to something else to be stable. The magnesium is "chelated" to organic and amino acids. The amount of magnesium in each supplement that can be assimilated by the digestive system and used for cellular activity is different with each type. Magnesium oxide, magnesium sulfate, and magnesium carbonate have a very low bioavailability rate, which is the degree at which it is absorbed. Magnesium glycinate, magnesium malate, and magnesium taurate are more bioavailable and have a variety of uses, but magnesium citrate is the best choice as a general supplement for those with oxalate issues.

Magnesium in magnesium citrate is relatively well-absorbed, and the citrate molecule has a direct inhibitory effect on the crystallization of calcium salts. In simple terms, this means that it will help prevent formation of calcium oxalate kidney stones. It will also help break down and release any stored oxalate. This may temporarily cause a variety of system wide pain and inflammation. Although a good thing, symptoms can sometimes become intense. Baking off the magnesium and increasing water intake will help eliminate the symptoms caused by the release of stored oxalates. Due to the laxative effects of magnesium citrate, diarrhea may occur when taken in excessive amounts. I believe it best to start magnesium citrate supplements low and slow. I started with 200 mg taken about an hour before my biggest meal of the day, which was dinner, and after determining it was well tolerated I started taking another 200 mg an hour before lunch. Magnesium citrate lowers stomach acid, similar to an antacid, so it's best to take it well in advance of a meal since stomach acids are needed to break down the meal. It's usually well tolerated on an empty stomach, so it could even be taken after a meal or at bedtime. If you can't tolerate magnesium citrate I would recommend taking magnesium taurate.

Eating a balanced diet is the key to maintaining good health and keeping your body in optimum condition. A balanced diet does not cut out food groups; it consists of a wide variety of foods. Most experts say that if you're eating a healthy diet you generally shouldn't need to take supplements. Sometimes an underlying health condition will interfere with your body's ability to absorb nutrients from your food.

BUILDING BLOCKS

There are many ways to give your body the building blocks it needs to restore health and rid itself of stored oxalates once the toxic burden is lessened. Despite the potential toxicity of even low levels of oxalates, our body is well equipped to deal with this food-born toxin if it is healthy and our detoxification pathways are not blocked. Improving detoxification pathways will help the body rid itself of toxins and release them from the tissues with greater speed and fewer symptoms. Even though oxalate crystals are hard and strong, they can dissolve and disappear. Our major detoxification pathways are the liver, intestines, kidneys, and skin.

The Liver Pathway

In order for the liver to detoxify it needs sulfur. Sulfur is a critical natural nutrient and one that is necessary for vibrant health and prevention of chronic diseases. It is the third most abundant mineral in the human body. Sulfur is present in every cell in the human body as well as a component of bones. It plays a critical role in detoxification as well as the production of gastrointestinal mucus. The mucus in our gastrointestinal track keeps our microbiome healthy, which in turn aids in oxalate metabolism.[30] Oxalates deplete your sulfur stores so you will need to restore this potent antioxidant. Insufficient amounts of sulfur in your body can cascade into a number of health problems as it will affect bones, joints, connective tissues, and more. To boost your body's level of sulfur, eat more cabbage, cauliflower, garlic, onions, broccoli, grass-fed beef, and organic free-range eggs. Eating sulfur rich foods flushes oxalates out of cells and helps stop oxalates from being absorbed. As a supplement, sulfur is available in two forms: dimethyl sulfoxide (DMSO) and methylsulfonylmethane (MSM). Both forms are commonly used as an alternative treatment for inflammation and joint pain. It's generally well tolerated and safe at dosages of up to four grams daily.

Another way to boost your body's level of sulfur, as well as raise levels of magnesium, is to soak in Epsom salt. Epsom salt is also known as magnesium sulfate. The magnesium and sulfate in the salts are absorbed into the body through the skin. Because the sulfur is already in the sulfate form, it does not need to be converted like other forms of sulfur do. One clinical study that was conducted by Rosemary Waring of the University of Birmingham in the United Kingdom states that blood and urine levels of magnesium and sulfate rose significantly after 19 test subjects were immersed in a warm bath of water and Epsom salt for 12 minutes.[31] The usual recommendation is to use 1 to 2 cups of Epsom salt to a tub of very warm water and soaking in it for about 5-12 minutes. Enjoying these salt soaks several times a week can maintain optimal levels of these minerals. Ingesting Epsom salt is sometimes recommended but that comes with risks such as severe stomach pain, nausea, vomiting, and bowel obstruction. Absorbing these minerals through the skin is the safest and easiest way to increase sulfate and magnesium in the body. Your body will absorb as much as it needs. Magnesium levels in the blood are tightly controlled. When blood reaches optimal levels of magnesium the urine levels will begin to rise. Your body needs sulfur to detoxify, but if you're excessively toxic, you'll have to go slow. If soaking makes you feel ill, discontinue your soaks for a while and resume when you are feeling better. The magnesium from Epsom salts baths that enters bodily tissues through the skin might also help to dissolve calcium oxalate crystals that have formed there.

The Intestinal Pathway

Intestinal support for detoxification and health should also be addressed. Probiotics have been found to protect the body from toxins, support immune function, make B vitamins, metabolize carcinogens, and ferment non-digestible fiber to increase nutrient absorption.[32] Probiotic supplementation or increased consumption of fermented foods such as yogurt, kefir, sauerkraut, and kimchi are generally regarded as necessary for restoring proper intestinal function, particularly if there is a past history of antibiotic use. A variety of live cultures are supplied by nature in fermented foods and drinks. Be aware, many of these fermented foods are now made using vinegar and high-heat pressure processing or pasteurization. These pickled foods are missing all the powerful probiotics and beneficial enzymes of traditionally fermented foods. Look for naturally fermented or live cultured products. These are most often found in the refrigerated section. Personally, I eat a variety of fermented foods and also take a 15 strain probiotic daily. The gastrointestinal track is colonized with a wide variety of bacterial species, some of which may have the ability to degrade oxalates reducing absorption. These species include numerous species of Lactobacillus and several species of Bifidobacteria. *Oxalobacter formigenes* is the only known oxalate-degrading species. These bacteria live in the large intestine where they rely on oxalates as their sole source of energy. So instead of the colon taking up oxalates that are later filtered out of the blood by the kidneys, *Oxalobacter formigenes* devours it, thereby minimizing the amount available for intestinal absorption and subsequent urinary excretion.[33] The prevalence of *Oxalobacter formigenes* in a population ranges from 38% to 62%, with colonization lowest in people susceptible to kidney stones and in people with greater antibiotic exposure, indicating that the bacterium may be particularly sensitive to antibiotics.[34]

A 2002 study on *Oxalobacter formigenes* and its potential role in human health revealed that Chloramphenicol, Clarithromycin (Biaxin), and Doxycycline antibiotics eradicate
this special oxalate-degrading microbe.[35] Those with a history of heavy or recent antibiotic use may be at much greater risk for oxalated related illness. No reliable methods of introducing *Oxalobacter formigenes* as a probiotic have been marketed as of yet. In November 2017, OxThera AB announced that it has been granted two new U.S. patents. They have previously been granted patents in Europe, Canada, China, Hong-Kong, India, and Japan. OxThera has the property rights to pharmaceutical compositions of *Oxalobacter Formigenes*, the oxalate degrading bacteria for the treatment of Hyperoxaluria and kidney stones. It's designed to break down dietary oxalates in the upper gastrointestinal tract.[36] Early stage clinical trials have begun. The drug will have to be tested and approved before the licensing stage.

Bone broth, also known as stock, is the hottest new health trend, but it's been around as long as humans have cooked with fire. It's simply simmering bones for hours in water. Today you find recipes that call for a small amount of vinegar to act as an acidic medium to leech out the minerals in the bones. This collagen and nutrient rich broth has a reputation for having incredible health benefits from improving joint health to healing the gastrointestinal tract. It has been shown to reduce inflammation and protect against gastric ulcers as well. Bone broth is rich in glutamine, arginine, hydroxyproline, and glycine. These amino acids are necessary to make collagen. When the bones of chicken, fish, or beef are simmered, the collagen in the bones, tendons, and joints form gelatin. Gelatin is what gives bone broth or stock its jelly-like consistency once it has cooled. Bone broth has become a staple of gut-healing diets. Nutritional analysis for an 8 ounce serving of bone broth is around 200 Calories, 17 grams of carbohydrates, 9 grams of fat and 16 grams of protein. It contains very small amounts of vitamins and minerals, except for 40% of the daily value for manganese, and about 30% of the daily value for vitamin C and B6.[37]

Bone broth should be included in the diet to give your body the nutrients it needs to heal itself from any damage oxalates may have caused. However, I must give a word of caution. Although bone broth is oxalate free, 12% of the amino acids in gelatin is hydroxyproline. Hydroxyproline is broken down in the liver and about 5-20% is excreted in the urine as oxalate. Ingestion of hydroxyproline increases urinary oxalates for a few hours after ingestion.[38] If you are prone to kidney stones, you should limit the amount of bone broth in your diet. To reap the health benefits, have an occasional cup of bone broth without any additional oxalate foods to your diet that day. Moderation is key. Oxalate levels in the blood are more tightly controlled and do not rise after the hydroxyproline has been broken down in the liver, which makesit safe if you are not prone to kidney stones.

Amino acids in gelatin, like all amino acids, can only be properly utilized when the diet contains sufficient fat-soluble vitamins found exclusively in animal fats. Therefore, don't hesitate to put cream or butter in your broth-based soups. You can get additional helpful amino acids such as glutamate and glutamine by adding foods such as red meat, poultry, broccoli, and cabbage to your bone broth. Glutamate is an amino acid that functions as a neurotransmitter and helps relay signals in your nervous system. The amino acid glutamine maintains normal function of the immune system, digestive system and the brain. Glutathione, which is made from a form of glutamate and other amino acids, helps your body absorb and use all other amino acids. It's the body's most important antioxidant. It is derived from several different amino acids and is absolutely essential to maintaining a healthy immune system.

Basic Method of Making Bone Broth

1. In a large stock pot, add bones and cover with water.
2. Bring the water to a boil, adding any vegetables or herbs.
3. Allow it to simmer several hours or overnight.
4. Strain out the bones and vegetables.
5. You can use the stock immediately, store it in the refrigerator for several days, or freeze it for several months.

The Kidney Pathway

Key nutrients to support and help detox your kidneys are arginine and citric acid from lemons. Arginine, also known as L-arginine, is a nutrient that's involved in a number of different functions in the body. It helps the kidneys remove waste products from the body and reduces the risk of oxalate damage and stone formation. It has been shown to protect the renal cells from oxidative injury.[39] Foods rich in L-arginine are dairy products and pumpkin seeds.

Lemons have particularly high concentrations of citric acid. Like magnesium and L-Arginine, citric acid protects cells from calcium oxalate crystal induced injury and helps prevent the formation of calcium oxalate stones.[40] It's also been proven to break up small stones that have started to form.

The Skin Pathway

Many studies demonstrate that toxins can also be eliminated through the skin, relieving the burden on the kidneys and liver. Oxalates have also been known to trap heavy metals such as mercury and lead in tissues.[41] Whether from exercise, steam baths, or traditional or infrared saunas, sweating cleanses the body of these metals along with many other toxins. Our skin is our largest organ so a significant amount of detoxification occurs through it. Exercise caution when starting any kind of sweat therapy. If you have high levels of toxins, you could go through feelings of illness as you detoxify. If you choose a steam bath or sauna, start out slowly and work your way up in the frequency of sessions as well as time spent per session. If you do not own a sauna and would like to try it, you can usually find them in most fitness centers.

CHAPTER SIX

HIGH MEDIUM AND LOW OXALATE FOODS

If you are advised to follow a low oxalate diet, the first thing you will want is a reliable list of foods and their oxalate content. An Internet search for oxalate content of foods lists will result in various lists but not a single compressive food list. When comparing lists you'll notice inconsistencies. Sometimes serving sizes are not even listed. Another issue with oxalate content of foods lists that creates questionable accuracy is the differing oxalate levels within the varieties of a food. For example, there are 2,500 varieties of apples grown the United States. Oxalate content in plants can vary due to differences in climate they were grown and the soil they were grown in. All of these issues can be very discouraging for the individual wishing to follow a low oxalate diet. This is one of the reasons why I wrote this book. My own research on reliable oxalate lists was extensive. I ended up with 4 separate lists that together make a fairly comprehensive list.

The first list is Harvard University's T. H. Chan School of Public Health Nutrition Department Oxalate Content of Foods List (2007).[42] This extensive list notes exact serving sizes, the oxalate category, and the oxalate value of each food. It is a very good list overall.

The second list I found valuable is from the Wichita Nephrology Group, P.A.[43] Their website has a large number of very helpful patient resources including low oxalate diet information along with an up to date (2017) oxalate food list. Although the list isn't comprehensive and exact serving sizes are omitted, this list is a very good guide for low, moderate, and high oxalate foods.

The third oxalate content of foods list comes from the University of Pittsburg Medical Center.[44] Exact serving sizes aren't listed but foods are categorized in low, moderate, and high oxalate groups. Many foods not found on other lists are listed here.

The fourth oxalate content of foods list comes from Dr. Ina Wong, Naturopathic Physician and Registered Acupuncturist in Victoria, BC, Canada.[45] Dr. Wong holds a Bachelor of Science in Biochemistry from University of Ottawa. All foods are measured at ½ cup servings unless otherwise indicated and are placed in categories of low, medium, and high oxalate groups.

As you will see in the following lists, they sometimes don't agree on oxalate levels of foods. Doing a cross comparison of foods and oxalate values on each list seemed necessary in order to settle discrepancies. Another noticeable difference in these lists is that foods are often listed in categories of low, medium, and high with no agreement on the oxalate values assigned to each category. Low seemed to average 0-4 mg, medium range averages 2-10 mg, and high averages range 7-12 mg. Very High ranges are from 11 mg upwards. For example, one list may place a food in a low category and another list will place that same food in the medium range even though the oxalate content in milligrams is the same. Knowing the food serving size and its exact measured amount of oxalate content for that serving is necessary to know the amount of oxalates you are consuming. The key to living low oxalate is to keep your daily oxalate consumption to 40-50 mg or less. As long as you are keeping count you can do this by choosing foods out of the low, medium and high oxalate range.

In a cross comparison of the four food lists considered most accurate, up to date, and rather extensive as a whole, I noticed some foods showed marked differences in oxalate content. For example, avocados are listed as high in one list but in the other three is listed as low. When three out of four agreed on an oxalate value, I accepted the most agreed upon value as correct. I added avocados to my diet without any oxalate issues.

In the following table foods with oxalate value discrepancies are listed with their oxalate content by list. My method for determining accuracy was to accept the values most lists agreed on.

Cross Comparison Listings of Foods with Varied Oxalate Results

Food	Serving Size	Harvard University's T.H. Chan School of Public Health Nutrition Department	Wichita Nephrology Group, P.A.	University of Pittsburg Medical Center.	Dr. Ina Wong, Naturopathic Physician and Registered Acupuncturist
Avocado	1	Very high 19 mg	Low	Low 0-2 mg	None
Blackberries	½ cup	Very low 2 mg	High		Very high 11 mg
Blueberries	½ cup	Very low 2 mg	High		Very high 11 mg
Strawberries	½ cup	Very low 2 mg	High	High 7 mg	High 10 mg
Kale	1 cup	Very low 2 mg	High	High 7 mg	High 10 mg
Mustard Greens	1 cup	Low 4 mg	High	High 7 mg	
Baked Potato	1	Very high 19 mg	Medium	Medium 2-6 mg	Medium 2-10 mg
Spaghetti	1 cup	High 11 mg	Low		Low 0-2 mg
White Rice	1 cup	High 11 mg	Low		Low 0-2 mg

Flour					
Graham Crackers	1	Very low 2 mg	High	High 7 mg ^	High 10 mg
Wheat Crackers	1	Very low 1 mg	High	High 7 mg ^	High 10 mg
All Purpose Flour	1 cup	Very high 17 mg	Medium	Medium 2-6 mg	Medium 2-10 mg
Cornmeal	1 cup	Very high 64 mg	Medium	Medium 2-6 mg	Medium 2-10 mg
Lentil Soup	1 cup	Very high 39 mg	Low	Low 0-2 mg	None
Coffee	8 oz.	Very low 1 mg	Medium	Medium 2-6 mg	Medium 2-10 mg

RESULTS:

Avocado - 1 Low 0-2 mg
Blackberries – ½ cup High 11 mg
Blueberries – ½ cup High 11 mg
Strawberries – ½ cup High 7-10 mg
Kale – 1 cup High 7-10 mg
Mustard Greens – 1 High 7 mg
cup Baked Potato – 1 Medium 2-10 mg
Spaghetti – 1 cup Low 0-2 mg
White Rice Flour – 1 cup Low 0-2 mg
Graham Crackers – 1 High 7-10 mg
All Purpose Flour – 1 cup Medium 2-10 mg
Cornmeal – 1 cup Medium 2-10 mg
Lentil Soup – 1 cup Low 0-2 mg
Coffee – 8 oz. Medium 2-10 mg

OXALATE CONTENT OF FOODS LISTS

List # 1
Harvard University's T. H. Chan School of Public Health Nutrition Department

Oxalate Content of Foods List

Food Group	Serving size	Oxalate Category	Oxalate Value
Fruits			
Whole Fruits			
Avocados	1 fruit	Very High	19 mg
Dates	1 date	Very High	24 mg
Grapefruit	1/2 fruit	Very High	12 mg
Kiwi	1 fruit	Very High	16 mg
Orange	1 fruit	Very High	29 mg
Raspberries	1 cup	Very High	48 mg
Tangerine	1 fruit	High	10 mg
Figs	1 medium fig	Moderate	9 mg
Apple Sauce	1 cup	Very Low	2 mg
Banana	1 fruit	Low	3 mg
Blackberries	1/2 cup	Very Low	2 mg
Blueberries	1/2 cup	Very Low	2 mg
Cherries	1 cup	Low	3 mg
Limes	1/2 fruit	Low	3 mg
Pears	1 fruit	Very Low	2 mg
Pineapple	1 cup	Low	4 mg
Strawberries	1/2 cup	Very Low	2 mg
Raisins	1 oz	Low	3 mg
Apples	1 fruit	Very Low	1 mg
Apricots	1 fruit	Little or None	0 mg
Cantaloupe	1/4 melon	Very Low	1 mg
Grapes	½ cup	Very Low	1 mg
Honeydew	1 cup	Very Low	1 mg
Lemons	1 wedge	Very Low	1 mg
Mango	1 fruit	Very Low	1 mg
Nectarine	1 fruit	Little or None	0 mg
Papaya	1 medium fruit	Very Low	1 mg
Peaches	1 fruit	Little or None	0 mg

Food Group	Serving size	Oxalate Category	Oxalate Value
Plantain	1 medium	Very Low	1 mg
Plums	1 fruit	Little or None	0 mg
Watermelon	1 slice	Very Low	1 mg
Canned Fruits			
Canned Pineapple	½ cup	Very High	24 mg
Canned Cherries	1/2 cup	Moderate	7 mg
Cranberry Sauce	1/2 cup	Very Low	2 mg
Canned Pears	1/2 cup	Very Low	1 mg
Canned Peaches	1/2 cup	Very Low	1 mg
Fruit Cocktail	1/2 cup	Very Low	1 mg
Dried Fruits			
Dried Figs	5 pieces/fruits	Very High	24 mg
Dried Pineapples	1/2 cup	Very High	30 mg
Dried Prunes	1/4 cup	High	11 mg
Dried Apples	1 cup	Very Low	2 mg
Dried Apricots	1 cup	Low	3 mg
Dried Cranberries	1/2 cup	Very Low	1 mg
Vegetables			
Bamboo Shoots	1 cup	Very High	35 mg
Beets	1/2 cup	Very High	76 mg
Fava Beans	1/2 cup	Very High	20 mg
Navy Beans	1/2 cup	Very High	76 mg
Okra	1/2 cup	Very High	57 mg
Olives	8-12 olives	Very High	18 mg
Parsnip	1/2 cup	Very High	15 mg
Kidney Beans	1/2 cup	Very High	15 mg
Refried Beans	1/2 cup	Very High	16 mg
Rhubarb	1/2 cup	Very High	541 mg
Rutabaga	1/2 cup	Very High	31 mg
Spinach, cooked	1/2 cup	Very High	755 mg
Spinach, raw	1 cup	Very High	656 mg
Tomato Sauce	1/2 cup	Very High	17 mg
Turnip, mashed	1/2 cup	Very High	30 mg
Yams, cubed	1/2 cup	Very High	40 mg
Carrots, raw	1/2 lg.	High	10 mg
Celery, cooked	1 cup	High	10 mg
Collards	1 cup	High	10 mg
Artichokes	1 small	Moderate	5 mg

High Medium and Low Oxalate Foods

Food Group	Serving size	Oxalate Category	Oxalate Value
Asparagus	4 spears	Moderate	6 mg
Carrots, cooked	1/2 cup	Moderate	7 mg
Hot Chili Pepper	1/2 cup	Moderate	5 mg
Mixed Vegetables, frozen	1/2 cup	Moderate	5 mg
Oriental vegetables, frozen	1/2 cup	Moderate	6 mg
Soybeans	1 cup	Moderate	7 mg
String Beans	1/2 cup	Moderate	9 mg
Tomato	1 med	Moderate	7 mg
Brussels Sprouts	1/2 cup	Very Low	2 mg
Celery, raw	1 stalk	Low	3 mg
Kale, chopped	1 cup	Very Low	2 mg
Mung Beans	1/2 cup	Low	3 mg
Mustard Greens	1 cup chopped	Low	4 mg
Sea Vegetables	1 cup	Low	3 mg
Alfalfa Sprouts	1/2 cup	Little or None	0 mg
Bok Choy	1 cup, raw	Very Low	1 mg
Broccoli, chopped	1/2 cup	Very Low	1 mg
Cabbage	1/2 cup	Very Low	1 mg
Cauliflower, cooked	1/2 cup	Very Low	1 mg
Chives	1 tsp	Little or None	0 mg
Corn	1/2 cup	Very Low	1 mg
Cucumber	1/4 cucumber	Very Low	1 mg
Endive	1/2 cup	Little or None	0 mg
Green Pepper	1 ring	Very Low	1 mg
Iceberg Lettuce	1 cup	Little or None	0 mg
Mushrooms	1 mushroom	Little or None	0 mg
Onions	1 small onion	Little or None	0 mg
Peas	1/2 cup	Very Low	1 mg
Pickles	1 pickle	Little or None	0 mg
Radish	10 count	Little or None	0 mg
Romaine Lettuce	1 cup	Little or None	0 mg
Scallions	1/2 cup	Very Low	1 mg
Sauerkraut	1/2 cup	Very Low	1 mg
Water Chestnuts	4 chestnuts	Little or None	0 mg
Yellow Squash	1/2 cup	Very Low	1 mg
Zucchini	1/2 cup	Very Low	1 mg

Food Group	Serving size	Oxalate Category	Oxalate Value
Potatoes			
French Fries	4 oz - 1/2 cup	Very High	97 mg
Baked Potato, with skin	1 medium	Very High	97 mg
Mashed Potatoes	1 cup	Very High	29 mg
Potato Chips	1 oz	Very High	21 mg
Potato Salad	1/3 cup	Very High	17 mg
Sweet Potatoes	1 cup	Very High	28 mg
Dairy			
Cream Products			
Homemade Cream Sauce	1 cup	Low	3 mg
Coffee Creamer	1 tbsp	Little or None	0 mg
Non-Dairy Creamer	1 tbsp	Little or None	0 mg
Sour Cream	1 tbsp	Little or None	0 mg
Ice Creams			
Ice Cream, vanilla	1/2 cup	Little or None	0 mg
Ice Cream, light	1/2 cup	Little or None	0 mg
Non Fat Ice Cream	1/2 cup	Little or None	0 mg
Yogurt			
Plain Yogurt	1 cup	Very Low	2 mg
Yogurt with Fruit	8 oz	Very Low	1 mg
Non Fat Fruit Yogurt	8 oz	Very Low	1 mg
Frozen Yogurt	1/2 cup	Very Low	1 mg
Low Fat Frozen Yogurt	1/2 cup	Very Low	1 mg
Cheese			
American Cheese	1 slice	Little or None	0 mg
Cheddar Cheese	1 slice	Little or None	0 mg
Low Fat Cheese	1 slice	Little or None	0 mg
Cottage Cheese	1/2 cup	Little or None	0 mg
Low Fat Cottage Cheese	1 cup	Little or None	0 mg

Food Group	**Serving size**	**Oxalate Category**	**Oxalate Value**
Cottage Cheese			
Fat Free	1/2 cup	Very Low	1 mg
Mozzarella	1 oz	Little or None	0 mg
Eggs			
Egg	1 medium	Little or None	0 mg
Egg Beaters	4 oz	Little or None	0 mg
Dairy Spreads			
Cream Cheese	1 oz	Little or None	0 mg
Cream Cheese, fat free	1 oz	Very Low	1 mg
Low Fat Cream Cheese	1 oz	Very Low	1 mg
Butter, salted	1 pat	Little or None	0 mg
Milk			
Chocolate Milk	1 cup	Moderate	7 mg
Powdered Milk	1 envelope	Low	3 mg
Fat Free Milk	1 cup	Very Low	1 mg
1% Milk	1 cup	Very Low	1 mg
2% Milk	1 cup	Very Low	1 mg
Whole Milk	1 cup	Very Low	1 mg
Buttermilk	1 cup	Very Low	1 mg
Breads & Grains			
Breads			
French Toast	2 slices	Very High	13 mg
English Muffin, Whole Wheat	1 muffin	High	12 mg
Pancakes homemade	4 cakes	High	11 mg
Pancakes (mix)	4 cakes	High	10 mg
Blueberry Muffins	1 muffin	Moderate	9 mg
Biscuits, plain or buttermilk	1 biscuit	Moderate	6 mg
Bran Muffins	1 muffin	Moderate	5 mg
Bran Muffin, low fat	1 muffin	Moderate	5 mg

Food Group	Serving size	Oxalate Category	Oxalate Value
Cracked Wheat Bread	1 slice	Moderate	5 mg
English Muffin	1 muffin	Moderate	8 mg
English Muffin, Multi-grain	1 muffin	Moderate	8 mg
English Muffin, Wheat	1 muffin	Moderate	7 mg
Low Fat Muffins	1 muffin	Moderate	5 mg
Rye Bread	1 slice	Moderate	7 mg
Tortillas, Corn	1 tortilla	Moderate	7 mg
Tortillas, Flour	1 tortilla	Moderate	8 mg
White Bread	1 slice	Moderate	5 mg
Wheat Bran Bread	1 slice	Moderate	7 mg
Whole Oat Bread	1 slice	Moderate	5 mg
Whole Wheat Bread	1 slice	Moderate	6 mg
Corn Bread	1 piece	Low	4 mg
Oatmeal Bread	1 piece	Low	4 mg
Oat Bran Muffin	1 small muffin	Low	4 mg
Oat Bran Bread	1 slice	Low	4 mg
Pastas, Rice & Grains			
Flour, All-Purpose	1 cup	Very High	17 mg
Brown Rice, cooked	1 cup	Very High	24 mg
Flour, Brown Rice	1 cup	Very High	65 mg
Buckwheat, Groats	1 cup cooked	Very High	133 mg
Bulgur, cooked	1 cup	Very High	86 mg
Corn Grits	1 cup	Very High	97 mg
Cornmeal	1 cup	Very High	64 mg
Couscous	1 cup	Very High	15 mg
Lasagna	1 serving	Very High	23 mg
Millet, cooked	1 cup	Very High	62 mg
Miso	1 cup	Very High	40 mg
Rice Bran	1 cup	Very High	281 mg
Soy Flour	1 cup	Very High	94 mg

Food Group	Serving size	Oxalate Category	Oxalate Value
Wheat Berries	1 cup cooked	Very High	98 mg
Wheat Flour, Whole Grain	1 cup	Very High	29 mg
Spaghetti	1 cup cooked	High	11 mg
White Rice Flour	1 cup	High	11 mg
Corn Flour	1 cup	Low	3 mg
Hummus	1 tbsp	Low	4 mg
Macaroni & Cheese	1 cup	Low	4 mg
White Rice, cooked	1 cup	Low	4 mg
Flour, Barley Malt	1 cup	Little or None	0 mg
Corn Bran	1 cup	Little or None	0 mg
Flaxseed	1 tbsp	Little or None	0 mg
Oat Bran, raw	1/3 cup	Little or None	0 mg

Meats & Fish

Meat and Meat Alternatives

Tofu	3.5 oz	Very High	13 mg
Veggie Burger	1 pattie	Very High	24 mg
Soy Burger	3.5 oz	High	12 mg
Chicken Nuggets	6 nuggets	Low	3 mg
Meatballs	2 meatballs	Very Low	2 mg
Turkey Dogs	1 dog	Low	3 mg
Antelope	3 oz	Little or None	0 mg
Bacon	2 slices	Little or None	0 mg
Bologna	1 slice	Little or None	0 mg
Buffalo	3 oz	Little or None	0 mg
Chicken Dog	1 dog	Very Low	1 mg
Chicken Liver	3 oz	Little or None	0 mg
Chicken	3 oz	Little or None	0 mg
Hot Dogs	1 dog	Very Low	1 mg
Ham	3 oz	Little or None	0 mg
Ground Beef	3 oz	Little or None	0 mg
Hamburger, lean (85%)	3 oz	Little or None	0 mg
Hamburger, Lean (75%)	3 oz	Little or None	0 mg
Hamburger, lean (90%)	3 oz	Very Low	1 mg

Food Group	Serving size	Oxalate Category	Oxalate Value
Liver	3.5 oz	Little or None	0 mg
Moose	3 oz	Little or None	0 mg
Pork	5 oz	Little or None	0 mg
Turkey	5 oz	Little or None	0 mg
Venison	3 oz	Little or None	0 mg
Wild Game Meat	3 oz	Very Low	1 mg
Fish			
Tuna Salad	1 cup	Moderate	6 mg
Fish Sticks, frozen	2 sticks	Low	3 mg
Crab, Alaskan King	3 oz	Little or None	0 mg
Bluefish	1 fillet	Very Low	1 mg
Clams, raw	3 oz	Little or None	0 mg
Cod, pacific	1 fillet	Little or None	0 mg
Cod Liver, Fish Oil	1 tsp	Little or None	0 mg
Flounder	3 oz	Little or None	0 mg
Haddock	3 oz	Little or None	0 mg
Halibut	3 oz	Little or None	0 mg
Herring, Atlantic & Pacific	3 oz	Very Low	1 mg
Mackerel	3 oz	Little or None	0 mg
Oysters	3 oz	Little or None	0 mg
Pollock	3 oz	Little or None	0 mg
Salmon, all types	4 oz	Little or None	0 mg
Sardines	3.75 oz	Little or None	0 mg
Shrimp	3 oz	Little or None	0 mg
Swordfish	1 piece	Little or None	0 mg
Tuna Fish, in oil	3.5 oz	Little or None	0 mg
Tuna Fish, in water	3.5 oz	Little or None	0 mg
Whiting	3 oz	Little or None	0 mg
Nuts and Seeds			
Almonds	1 oz	Very High	122 mg
Candies, with nuts (Snickers)	2 oz	Very High	38 mg

Food Group	Serving size	Oxalate Category	Oxalate Value
Cashews	1 oz	Very High	49 mg
Peanuts	1 oz	Very High	27 mg
Pistachios	1 oz	Very High	14 mg
Mixed Nuts, with peanuts	1 oz	Very High	39 mg
Pumpkin Seeds	1 cup, cooked	Very High	17 mg
Trail Mix	1 oz	Very High	15 mg
Walnuts	1 cup	Very High	31 mg
Pecans	1 oz	High	10 mg
Sunflower Seeds	1 cup	High	12 mg
Flaxseed	1 tbsp	Little or None	0 mg
Cakes, Candies Cookies & Pudding Snacks			
Brownies	1 oz	Very High	31 mg
Cake, store brand	1 piece	Very High	15 mg
Cake, homemade	1 piece	Very High	16 mg
Chocolate Syrup	2 tbsp	Very High	38 mg
Fudge Sauce	2 tbsp	Very High	28 mg
Cake, low fat only	1 piece	High	11 mg
Chocolate Chip Cookie	1 cookie	High	10 mg
Milk Chocolate Candies	1 oz	Moderate	5 mg
Apple Pie	1(1/8th) piece	Moderate	5 mg
Pudding Popsicle	1 popsicle	Moderate	5 mg
Fig Bars	1 cookie	Low	4 mg
Chocolate Pudding, Instant	1 oz or 1/4 box	Low	4 mg
Oatmeal Cookies	1 cookie	Low	4 mg
Rice Cake	1 cake	Low	4 mg
Rice Pudding	1/2 cup	Very Low	2 mg
Snack Cakes, crème filled	1 cake	Low	3 mg
Custard	1 cup	Very Low	1 mg
Jell-O	1 cup	Very Low	1 mg
Popsicle	1 stick	Little or None	0 mg
Rice Krispy Treat	1 bar	Very Low	1 mg
Sherbet	1/2 cup	Little or None	0 mg

Food Group	Serving size	Oxalate Category	Oxalate Value
Tapioca Pudding	1/2 cup	Little or None	0 mg
Vanilla Pudding	1 cup	Very Low	1 mg
Crackers, Chips and Miscellaneous			
Potato Chips	1 oz	Very High	21 mg
Tortilla Corn Chips	1 oz	Moderate	7 mg
Popcorn, oil-popped	1 cup	Moderate	5 mg
Pretzels, hard salted	1 oz	Moderate	5 mg
Fruit Roll-Ups	1 roll	Very Low	2 mg
Graham Crackers	1 large rectangle	Very Low	2 mg
Popcorn, air-popped	1 cup	Low	4 mg
Ritz Crackers	5 crackers	Low	3 mg
Saltines	1 cracker	Very Low	1 mg
Triscuits	1 cracker	Very Low	1 mg
Wheat Crackers	1 cracker	Very Low	1 mg
Wheat Thins, Reduced Fat	1 cracker	Very Low	1 mg
Beverages			
Carrot Juice	1 cup	Very High	27 mg
Hot Chocolate, homemade	1 cup	Very High	65 mg
Lemonade, frozen concentrate	8 oz	Very High	15 mg
Rice Dream	1 cup	Very High	13 mg
Tea, brewed	1 cup	Very High	14 mg
Tomato Juice	1 cup	Very High	14 mg
V8 Juice	1 cup	Very High	18 mg
Prune Juice	1 cup	Moderate	7 mg
Apple Juice	6 oz	Very Low	2 mg
Apricot Juice	1 cup	Very Low	2 mg
Coffee, decaff	1 cup	Very Low	2 mg
Orange Juice	1 cup	Very Low	2 mg
Pineapple Juice	8 oz	Low	3 mg

Food Group	Serving size	Oxalate Category	Oxalate Value
Postum, coffee Substitute	1 serving	Very Low	2 mg
Coffee	1 cup	Very Low	1 mg
Gatorade	1 cup	Little or None	0 mg
Grape Juice	8 oz	Very Low	1 mg
Grapefruit Juice	8 oz	Little or None	0 mg
Kool-Aid	1 cup	Very Low	1 mg
Lemonade, diet	8 oz	Very Low	1 mg
Mango Juice	8 oz	Very Low	1 mg
Sodas (all types)	8 oz	Little or None	0 mg
Sweetened Instant Iced Tea	1 cup	Little or None	0 mg
Water	8 oz	Little or None	0 mg
Dairy Beverages			
Chocolate Milk	1 cup	Moderate	7 mg
Powdered Milk	1 envelope	Low	3 mg
Soy Milk	1 cup	Low	4 mg
Fat Free Milk	1 cup	Very Low	1 mg
1% Milk	1 cup	Very Low	1 mg
2% Milk	1 cup	Very Low	1 mg
Whole Milk	1 cup	Very Low	1 mg
Alcoholic Beverages			
Beer, regular	1 can	Low	4 mg
Red Wine	4 oz	Very Low	1 mg
Beer, light	1 can	Low	3 mg
White Wine	4 oz	Little or None	0 mg
Liquor, 80 proof	1 jigger	Little or None	0 mg
Spread, Sauces & Toppings			
Fudge Sauce	2 tbsp	Very High	28 mg
Chocolate Syrup	2 tbsp	Very High	38 mg
Miso	1 cup	Very High	40 mg
Peanut Butter	1 tbsp	Very High	13 mg
Peanut Butter, Reduced fat	1 tbsp	Very High	16 mg
Stuffing	1 cup	Very High	36 mg

Food Group	Serving size	Oxalate Category	Oxalate Value
Tahini	1 tbsp	Very High	16 mg
Cream Sauce	1 cup	Low	3 mg
Gravy	1 cup	Low	4 mg
Olive Oil & Vinegar		Very Low	2 mg
Soy Sauce	1 tbsp	Low	3 mg
Apple Butter	1 tbsp	Little or None	0 mg
Butter	1 pat	Little or None	0 mg
Catsup/Ketchup	1 packet	Very Low	1 mg
Cream Cheese	1 oz	Little or None	0 mg
Cream Cheese, low fat	1 oz	Very Low	1 mg
Cream Cheese, fat free	1 oz	Very Low	1 mg
Horseradish	1 tbsp	Little or None	0 mg
Jam/Jelly	1 tbsp	Very Low	1 mg
Italian Salad Dressing	1 tbsp	Little or None	0 mg
Mayonnaise	1 tbsp	Little or None	0 mg
Mustard, yellow	1 tsp	Very Low	1 mg
Pancake Syrup	3/4 tbsp	Little or None	0 mg
Salsa	1 tbsp	Very Low	1 mg
Whipped Cream	2 tbsp	Little or None	0 mg
Whipped Topping	2 tbsp	Little or None	0 mg
Ingredients			
Flour, All-Purpose	1 cup	Very High	17 mg
Flour, Brown Rice	1 cup	Very High	65 mg
Cocoa Powder	4 tsp	Very High	67 mg
Cornmeal	1 cup	Very High	64 mg
Soy Flour	1 cup	Very High	94 mg
Soy Protein Isolate	1 oz	Very High	27 mg
Wheat Flour, whole grain	1 cup	Very High	29 mg
Flour, white rice	1 cup	High	11 mg
Chili Powder	1 tbsp	Moderate	7 mg

Food Group	Serving size	Oxalate Category	Oxalate Value
Brewer's Yeast	1 tbsp	Moderate	7 mg
Corn Flour	1 cup	Low	3 mg
Cornstarch	1 cup	Low	3 mg
Lemon Juice, can or bottle	1 cup	Low	4 mg
Artificial Sweetener	1 packet	Very Low	1 mg
Bouillon Cube	1 cube	Very Low	1 mg
Black Pepper	1 dash	Little or None	0 mg
Flour, barley malt	1 cup	Little or None	0 mg
Brown Sugar	1 cup packed	Very Low	1 mg
Butter	1 pat	Little or None	0 mg
Buttermilk	1 cup	Very Low	1 mg
Corn Syrup, high fructose	1 tbsp	Very Low	1 mg
Corn Syrup, Light	1 tbsp	Little or None	0 mg
Cod Liver Oil	1 tsp	Little or None	0 mg
Cream Substitute	1 tsp	Little or None	0 mg
Cream	1 tbsp	Little or None	0 mg
Eggs	1 medium egg	Little or None	0 mg
Eggbeaters	4 oz	Little or None	0 mg
Garlic Powder	1 tsp	Little or None	0 mg
Gelatin	1 tbsp	Little or None	0 mg
Honey	1 tbsp	Little or None	0 mg
Lard	1 tsp	Little or None	0 mg
Lemon Juice, raw	1 tbsp	Little or None	0 mg
Molasses	1 tbsp	Little or None	0 mg
Oat Flour	1 cup	Little or None	0 mg
Salt	1 tsp	Little or None	0 mg
Shortening	1 tsp	Little or None	0 mg
Sugar	1 tsp	Little or None	0 mg
Sweet Whey, fluid	1 cup	Very Low	1 mg
Sweet Whey, dried	1 tbsp	Little or None	0 mg

Food Group	Serving size	Oxalate Category	Oxalate Value
Fast Food Items Or Meals			
Cheeseburger, with bun	1 burger	Very High	13 mg
Burritos, with beans	1 burrito	Very High	17 mg
Burritos, with beans & meat	1 burrito	Very High	16 mg
Chili with Beans	1 cup	Very High	24 mg
Enchilada, beef & cheese	1 enchilada	Very High	13 mg
Enchilada, with chicken	1 enchilada	Very High	13 mg
French Fries	4 oz	Very High	51 mg
Lasagna, with meat	1 serving	Very High	23 mg
Nachos, with cheese	6-8 chips	Very High	13 mg
Cheese Pizza	2 slices	Very High	13 mg
Grilled Cheese	1 sandwich	High	12 mg
Tacos	1 small taco	High	12 mg
Doughnut	1 doughnut	Moderate	5 mg
Eggroll	1 eggroll	Moderate	5 mg
Hot Dog, with bun	1 dog with bun	Moderate	9 mg
Onion Rings	6-8 rings	Moderate	5 mg
Chicken Nuggets	6 nuggets	Low	3 mg
Macaroni & Cheese	1 cup	Low	4 mg
Chicken Roll	1 package	Very Low	1 mg
Soups			
Clam Chowder	1 cup	Very High	13 mg
Lentil Soup	1 cup	Very High	39 mg
Miso Soup	1 cup	Very High	111 mg
Vegetable Beef Soup	1 cup	Moderate	5 mg
Chicken Noodle Soup	1 can	Low	3 mg

Food Group	Serving size	Oxalate Category	Oxalate Value
Breakfast Items			
Cream of Wheat	1 cup	Very High	18 mg
Red River Cereal	1/4 cup	Very High	13 mg
Corn Grits	1 cup	Very High	97 mg
Farina Cereal	1 cup	Very High	16 mg
French Toast	2 slices	Very High	13 mg
Pancakes, homemade	4 pancakes	Very High	22 mg
Pancakes, dry mix	4 pancakes	Very High	37 mg
Danish Pastry, homemade	1 pastry	Very High	14 mg
Sweet Rolls, low fat	1 pastry	Very High	13 mg
English Muffins, whole wheat	1 muffin	High	12 mg
Bran Muffins	1 muffin	Moderate	5 mg
Bran Muffin, low fat	1 muffin	Moderate	5 mg
Muffin, blueberry	1 muffin	Moderate	9 mg
Doughnut	1 doughnut	Moderate	5 mg
English Muffins	1 muffin	Moderate	8 mg
English Muffins, multi-grain	1 muffin	Moderate	8 mg
English Muffins, wheat	1 muffin	Moderate	7 mg
Muffins, low fat	1 muffin	Moderate	5 mg
Poptart	1 tart	Moderate	7 mg
Cornbread	1 piece	Low	4 mg
Danish Pastry, fruit filled	1 pastry	Low	4 mg
Granola Bars, low fat	1 oz uncoated	Very Low	2 mg
Kashi Go Lean Bar	1 bar	Low	3 mg
Carnation Instant Breakfast	1 packet	Very Low	1 mg
Bacon	2 slices	Little or None	0 mg
Eggs	1 medium egg	Little or None	0 mg
Eggbeaters	4 oz	Little or None	0 mg

Food Group	Serving size	Oxalate Category	Oxalate Value
Granola Bars, hard & plain	1 bar	Very Low	1 mg
Oatmeal Cereal	1 cup	Little or None	0 mg
Pancake Syrup	3/4 tbsp	Little or None	0 mg

Cereals by Manufacturer

Kellogg's

Food Group	Serving size	Oxalate Category	Oxalate Value
All-Bran Original	1/2 cup	Very High	26 mg
All-Bran Buds	1/2 cup	Very High	20 mg
Complete Wheat Bran	3/4 cup	Very High	34 mg
Cracklin' Oat Bran	3/4 cup	Very High	15 mg
Frosted Mini-Wheat	1 cup	Very High	28 mg
Just Right Fruit & Nut	1 cup	Very High	13 mg
Low Fat Granola, with Raisins	2/3 cup	Very High	16 mg
Kashi Go Lean	3/4 cup	Very High	14 mg
Mueslix Apple & Almond	2/3 cup	Very High	20 mg
Mueslix	2/3 cup	Very High	17 mg
Puffed Kashi	1 cup	Very High	13 mg
Raisin Bran	1 cup	Very High	46 mg
Raisin Bran Crunch	1 cup	Very High	27 mg
Raisin Squares Mini-Wheat	1 cup	Very High	41 mg
Smart Start	1 cup	Very High	15 mg
All-Bran with extra fiber	1/2 cup	High	11 mg
Cocoa Krispies	3/4 cup	High	11 mg
Kashi Good Friends	3/4 cup	High	10 mg
Complete Oat Bran Flakes	3/4 cup	Moderate	5 mg
Kashi Heart to Heart	3/4 cup	Moderate	8 mg
Healthy Choice multi-grain	3/4 cup	Moderate	7 mg
Froot Loops	1 cup	Very Low	2 mg

Food Group	Serving size	Oxalate Category	Oxalate Value
Honey Crunch Corn Flakes	3/4 cup	Low	3 mg
Rice Krispies	1 1/4 cup	Low	4 mg
Special K	1 cup	Low	3 mg
Special K Red Berries	1 cup	Very Low	2 mg
Smacks	3/4 cup	Low	3 mg
Corn Flakes	1 cup	Very Low	1 mg
Corn Pops	1 cup	Very Low	1 mg
Crispix	1 cup	Very Low	1 mg
Frosted Flakes	3/4 cup	Very Low	1 mg
Product 19	1 cup	Very Low	1 mg
Post Cereals			
100% Bran	1/3 cup	Very High	25 mg
40% Bran	3/4 cup	Very High	36 mg
Banana Nut Crunch	1 cup	Very High	25 mg
Cranberry Almond Crunch	1 cup	Very High	35 mg
Fruit & Fiber Dates	1 cup	Very High	41 mg
Great Grains Raisin, Dates, Pecans	1 cup	Very High	17 mg
Grape Nuts	1/2 cup	Very High	14 mg
Shredded Wheat & Bran	1 1/4 cup	Very High	53 mg
Blueberry Morning	1/2 cup	Moderate	8 mg
Grape Nuts Flakes	3/4 cup	Moderate	7 mg
Fruity Pebbles	3/4 cup	Very Low	2 mg
Honeycomb	1 1/3 cup	Very Low	1 mg
Wafflecrisp	1 cup	Very Low	1 mg
General Mills			
Basic 4	1 cup	Very High	17 mg
Fiber One	1/2 cup	Very High	13 mg
Honey Nut Clusters	1 cup	Very High	23 mg
Multi-Bran Chex	1 cup	Very High	36 mg

Food Group	Serving size	Oxalate Category	Oxalate Value
Nature Valley Cinnamon Raisin Granola	3/4 cup	Very High	13 mg
Oatmeal Crisp with Almonds	1 cup	Very High	24 mg
Oatmeal Raisin Crisp	1 cup	Very High	13 mg
Raisin Nut Bran	1 cup	Very High	24 mg
Total Raisin Bran	1 cup	Very High	31 mg
Harmony	1 1/4 cup	High	11 mg
Wheaties Raisin Bran	1 cup	High	11 mg
Apple Cinnamon Cheerios	3/4 cup	Moderate	5 mg
Berry Bust Cheerios	1 cup	Moderate	7 mg
Cheerios	1 cup	Moderate	8 mg
Cinnamon Toast Crunch	3/4 cup	Moderate	5 mg
Corn Chex	1 cup	Moderate	5 mg
Count Chocula	1 cup	Moderate	5 mg
Frosted Cheerios	1 cup	Moderate	6 mg
Honey Nut Cheerios	1 cup	Moderate	7 mg
Golden Grahams	3/4 cup	Moderate	9 mg
Lucky Charms	1 cup	Moderate	5 mg
Reese's Puffs	3/4 cup	Moderate	8 mg
Team Cheerios	1 cup	Moderate	6 mg
Total Corn Flakes	1 1/3 cup	Moderate	5 mg
Wheat Chex	1 cup	Moderate	7 mg
Wheaties	1 cup	Moderate	8 mg
Whole Grain Total	3/4 cup	Moderate	8 mg
Cocoa Puffs	1 cup	Low	3 mg
Kix	1 1/3 cup	Very Low	2 mg
Rice Chex	1 1/4 cup	Low	4 mg
Trix	1 cup	Little or None	0 mg
Quaker			
Low Fat 100% Natural Granola with Raisins	3/4 cup	Very High	15 mg

Food Group	Serving size	Oxalate Category	Oxalate Value
100% Natural Granola			
Oats and Honey	1/2 cup	Very High	13 mg
Oat Bran	1 1/4 cup	High	10 mg
Honey Nut Oats	1 oz	Moderate	7 mg
Oatmeal Squares	1 cup	Moderate	5 mg
Puffed Wheat	1 1/4 cup	Moderate	9 mg
Toasted Oatmeal	1 oz	Moderate	6 mg
Puffed Rice	1 cup	Very Low	2 mg
Qaker Oat Cinnamon Life	3/4 cup	Low	3 mg
Quaker Oat Life	3/4 cup	Low	3 mg
Cap'n Crunch	3/4 cup	Little or None	0 mg
Other Cereal Brands			
Bran Flakes with Raisins, Single Brand	1 cup	Very High	57 mg
Nabisco Shredded Wheat	2 biscuits	Very High	42 mg
Nabisco Honey Nut Shredded Wheat, Bite Sized	1 cup	Very High	47 mg
Spoonsize Shredded Wheat	1 cup	Very High	45 mg
Uncle Sam	1 cup	High	11 mg
Just Right with Crunchy Nuggcts	1 cup	Moderate	5 mg
Wheetabix Whole Wheat	2 biscuits	Moderate	8 mg
Healthy Valley Oat Bran Flakes	1 cup	Little or None	0 mg

List # 2

Wichita Nephrology Group, P.A.

Low Oxalate Diet

Drinks

Low Oxalate	Moderate Oxalate	High Oxalate
apple juice	coffee (limit to 8 oz/day)	any juice made from high oxalate fruits
beer, bottled or canned	cola (limit to 12 oz/day)	beer, draft
cider	cranberry juice	chocolate, plain*
distilled alcohol	grape juice	chocolate milk
ginger ale	orange juice	cocoa*
grapefruit juice	orangeade	coffee powder (instant)*
lemon juice		Ovaltine
lemonade/limeade (made without peel)		tea, brewed*
lime juice		
milk (skim, 2%, whole)		
orange soda		
pineapple		
root beer		
tea, instant		
water		
wine		

Dairy

Low Oxalate	Moderate Oxalate	High Oxalate
milk (skim, 2%, whole)	none	chocolate milk
buttermilk		
yogurt with allowed fruit		
cheese		
For calcium restrictions, limit above to one serving per day.		

Meat

Low Oxalate	Moderate Oxalate	High Oxalate
beef, lamb, pork	beef kidney	none
eggs	liver	
fish/shellfish		
poultry		

Meat Substitutes, Beans, Nuts, and Seeds

Low Oxalate	Moderate Oxalate	High Oxalate
eggs	garbanzo beans, canned	almonds
lentils	lima beans	baked beans canned in tomato sauce
water chestnuts	split peas, cooked	cashews
		green beans, waxed and dried
		peanut butter*
		peanuts*

Low Oxalate	Moderate Oxalate	High Oxalate
		pecans*
		sesame seeds
		sunflower seeds
		tofu (soybean curd)*
		walnuts

** This food is extremely high in oxalates, 7 to 700 mg per serving*

Fruit

Low Oxalate	Moderate Oxalate	High Oxalate
apples, peeled	apples with skin	blackberries
avocado	apricots	black raspberries*
bananas	black currants	blueberries
cantaloupe	cranberries, dried	red currants
casaba	grapefruit	dewberries
cherries, bing	oranges	figs, dried
coconut	peaches	grapes, purple
cranberries, canned	pears	gooseberries
grapes, green	pineapple	kiwi
honeydew	plums	lemon peel*
mangoes	prunes	lime peel*
nectarines		orange peel
papaya		red raspberries
raisins		rhubarb*
watermelon		strawberries
		tangerines

Low Oxalate	Moderate Oxalate	High Oxalate
		any juice made from above fruits

** This food is extremely high in oxalates, 7 to 700 mg per serving*

Breads and Starches

Low Oxalate	Moderate Oxalate	High Oxalate
bread	barley, cooked	Fig Newtons
breakfast cereals	corn bread	fruit cake
noodles, egg or macaroni	corn tortilla	graham crackers
ice, white or wild	cornmeal	grits, white corn
	cornstarch	kamut
	flour, white or wheat	marmalade
	oatmeal	soybean crackers*
	rice, brown	wheat germ*
	unsalted saltine or soda crackers	
	spaghetti in tomato sauce	
	sponge cake	

** This food is extremely high in oxalates, 7 to 700 mg per serving*

Vegetables

Low Oxalate	Moderate Oxalate	High Oxalate
acorn squash	asparagus	beans (green, wax, dried)

Low Oxalate	Moderate Oxalate	High Oxalate
alfalfa sprouts	artichokes	beets (tops, roots, greens)
cabbage	brussels sprouts	celery
cauliflower	broccoli	chives
peas, frozen and fresh	carrots	collards
peppers, red	corn	dandelion
radishes	cucumbers, peeled	eggplant
turnips, roots	kohlrabi	escarole
zucchini	lettuce	kale
squash	lima beans	leeks*
	mushrooms	mustard greens
	onions	okra*
	potatoes, white	parsley
	peas, canned	parsnips
	snow peas	peppers, green
	tomato, fresh	pokeweed*
	tomato sauce	rutabagas
		sorrel
		spinach*
		summer squash
		sweet potatoes*
		Swiss chard*
		tomato soup
		vegetable soup

Low Oxalate	Moderate Oxalate	High Oxalate
		watercress
		yams

** This food is extremely high in oxalates, 7 to 700 mg per serving*

Condiments

Low Oxalate	Moderate Oxalate	High Oxalate
any not listed	basil, fresh	cinnamon, ground
	malt, powder	parsley, raw*
	pepper	pepper, more than 1 tsp/day*
		ginger
		soy sauce

** This food is extremely high in oxalates, 7 to 700 mg per serving*

Wichita Nephrology Group, P.A. 2017

818 N Emporia, Suite 310, Wichita, KS 67214

List #3
University of Pittsburgh Medical Center

Low Oxalate Diet

Low Oxalate	Moderate Oxalate	High Oxalate
Drinks		
apple juice-	coffee (limit to 8 oz/day)	any juice from high-oxalate fruits
beer, bottled or canned	cola (limit to 12 oz/day)	beer, draft
cider	cranberry juice-	chocolate, plain*
distilled alcohol	grape juice	chocolate milk
ginger ale	orange juice	cocoa*
grapefruit juice	orangeade	coffee powder
(instant)*		
lemon juice		Ovaltine
lemonade/limeade-made without peel)		tea, brewed*
lime juice		
milk (skim, 2%, whole)		
orange soda		
pineapple		
root beer		
tea, instant		
water		
wine		
Dairy		
milk (skim, 2%, whole)	none	chocolate milk
buttermilk		
yogurt		
cheese		

Low Oxalate	Moderate Oxalate	High Oxalate
Meat		
beef, lamb, pork	beef kidney	none
eggs	liver	
fish/shellfish		
poultry		
Meat Substitutes, Beans, Nuts, and Seeds		
eggs	garbanzo beans, canned	almonds
lentils	lima beans	baked beans canned in tomato sauce
water chestnuts	split peas, cooked	cashews
		green beans, waxed and dried
		peanut butter*
		peanuts*
		pecans*
		sesame seeds
		sunflower seeds
		tofu (soybean curd)*
		walnuts
Fats and Oils		
All	none	none
Breads and Starches		
bread	barley, cooked	Fig Newtons
breakfast cereals	corn bread	fruit cake
noodles, egg or macaroni	corn tortilla	graham crackers
rice, white or wild	cornmeal	grits, white corn
	cornstarch	kamut
	flour, white or wheat	marmalade
	oatmeal	soybean crackers
	rice, brown	wheat germ*

Low Oxalate	Moderate Oxalate	High Oxalate
	unsalted saltine	
	or soda crackers	
	spaghetti in tomato sauce	
	sponge cake	
Fruit		
apples, peeled	apples with skin	blackberries
avocado	apricots	black
raspberries*		
bananas	black currants	blueberries
cantaloupe	cranberries, dried	red currants
casaba	grapefruit	dewberries
cherries, bing	oranges	figs, dried
coconut	peaches	grapes, purple
cranberries, canned	pears	gooseberries
grapes, green	pineapple	kiwi
honeydew	plums	lemon peel*
mangoes	prunes	lime peel*
nectarines		orange peel
papaya		red raspberries
raisins		rhubarb*
watermelon		strawberries
		tangerines
		any juice made
		from above
		fruits
Vegetables		
acorn squash	asparagus	beans (green,
wax, dried)		
alfalfa sprouts	artichokes	beets (top, root,
		greens)
cabbage	Brussels sprouts	celery
cauliflower	broccoli	chives
peas, frozen and fresh	carrots	collards
peppers, red	corn	dandelion

Low Oxalate	Moderate Oxalate	High Oxalate
radishes	cucumbers, peeled	eggplant
turnips, roots	kohlrabi	escarole
zucchini	lettuce	kale
squash	lima beans	leeks*
	mushrooms	mustard greens
	onions	okra*
	potatoes, white	parsley
	peas, canned	parsnips
	snow peas	peppers, green
	tomato, fresh	pokeweed*
	tomato sauce	rutabagas
		sorrel
		spinach*
		summer squash
		sweet potatoes*
		Swiss chard*
		tomato soup
		vegetable soup
		watercress
Condiments		
any not listed	basil, fresh	cinnamon, ground
	malt, powder	parsley, raw*
	pepper	pepper, more than 1 tsp/day*
		ginger
		soy sauce

* This food is extremely high in oxalates, 7 to 700 mg. per serving.

All serving sizes are 1/2 cup unless otherwise indicated.

List #4

Dr. Ina Wong, Naturopathic Physician and Registered Acupuncturist

Oxalate Content of Foods

Little or no oxalates (< 2 mg per serving)	**Moderate oxalates** (2-10 mg per serving) Limit to 2 servings a day	**High oxalates** (> 10 mg per serving) Avoid
Beverages:		
Apple juice	Coffee	Draft beer, stout,
Guinness, draft		
Grapefruit juice	Cranberry juice	lager, Tuborg, Pilsner
Lemonade, limeade (no peel)	Grape juice	Juices containing berries
Pineapple juice	Orange juice	Ovaltine & other beverage
mixes		
Distilled alcohol	Tomato juice	Tea
Wine (port, red, rose, white)	Nescafe powder (1 cup)	Cocoa
Cider	Beer	Chocolate milk
Milk	Orangeade	Black Indian tea
Bigelow herbal teas:	V-8 juice	Bigelow herbal teas:
• Cozy chamomile	Wine (Beaujolais)	• Apple orchard
• Purely peppermint	Bigelow herbal teas:	• Fruit & almond
• Apple & spice	•Lemon & C	• I love lemon
• Chamomile mint	• Spearmint	• Mint medley
• Cinnamon orange		• Orange spice
• Hibiscus & rose hips		• Perfect peach
• Tahitian breeze		• Red raspberry
Water		• Specially strawberry
		• Sweet dreams
		• Take a Break
		• Orange & C
Condiments:		
Chives	Basil (1 tbsp)	Cinnamon (> 1 1/2 tsp)
Mustard, Dijon (1 tbsp)	Dill (1 tbsp)	Pepper (> 1 tsp)
Nutmeg (1 tsp)	Cinnamon (1 tsp)	Ginger (1 tbsp)
Oregano (1 tsp)	Ginger (1 tsp)	Soy sauce
Salt	Malt powder (1 tbsp)	
Vanilla extract	Mustard, Dijon (1/2 cup)	

High Medium and Low Oxalate Foods

Little or no oxalates (< 2 mg per serving)	**Moderate oxalates** (2-10 mg per serving) Limit to 2 servings a day	**High oxalates** (> 10 mg per serving) Avoid
Vinegar (not fruit on high list)	Nutmeg (1 tbsp)	
	Pepper (1 tsp)	
Meats:		
Beef	Bacon (> 10 slices)	
Poultry	Kidney, beef	
Eggs	Liver	
Fish	Sardines	
Pork		
Lamb		
Dairy:		
Butter		
Buttermilk		
Cheese		
Milk		
Yoghurt (check fruits on high list)		
Mayonnaise		
Grains:		
Cornflakes	Corn bread	Whole wheat bread
Cornstarch (1 tbsp)	Sponge cake	Cheerios
Egg noodles	Spaghetti with tomato sauce	Graham crackers
White rice		Soda crackers
Grits	Cornstarch (1/4 cup)	Kamut
Wild rice	Corn tortilla	Oatmeal
Brown rice	Cornmeal (1 cup)	Popcorn (4 cups)
Rye	Wheat flour	Soybean cracker
Spaghetti		Spelt
		Stone ground flour
		Wheat bran
		Wheat germ
		Whole wheat flour
Fruits:		
Apples, peeled	Apples, with peel	Blackberries
Avocado	Apricots	Blueberries
Bananas	Cherries (red, sour)	Dewberries
Cherries (Bing)	Cranberries, dried	Gooseberries
Cranberries	Grapefruit	Raspberries
Grapes (Thompson seedless, green, red)	Grapes (except Thompson seedless green, red)	Strawberries
		Grapes (Concord)

Little or no oxalates (< 2 mg per serving)	**Moderate oxalates** (2-10 mg per serving) Limit to 2 servings a day	**High oxalates** (> 10 mg per serving) Avoid
Lemons	Oranges	Currants
Limes	Peaches	Figs
Mangoes	Pears	Kiwi
Melons	Pineapple	Lemon, lime, orange peel
Cantaloupe	Plums	Rhubarb
Honeydew	Prunes	
Water melon	Tangerines	
Nectarines		
Papaya		
Vegetables:		
Brussels sprouts	Asparagus	Beets (root, greens)
Cauliflower	Artichokes	Celery
Cabbage	Broccoli	Collards
Radish	Carrots	Dandelion greens
Alfalfa sprouts	Corn	Eggplant
Cucumbers, peeled	Garlic	Escarole
Red pepper	Green peas	Beans (green, snap, pod, runner)
Turnip	Kohlrabi	Kale
Zucchini	Lettuce (butter, iceburg)	Leeks
	Mushrooms	Okra
	Mustard greens	Parsley
	Green peppers	Parsnips
	Onions	Potatoes
	Potatoes (white, russet)	Sweet potatoes
	Snow peas	Pumpkin
	Tomato	Rhubarb
	Watercress	Rutabaga
		Sorrel
		Spinach
		Squash (yellow, summer)
		Swiss chard
		Tomato sauce, (canned)
		Turnip greens
		Yams

Little or no oxalates (< 2 mg per serving)	**Moderate oxalates** (2-10 mg per serving) Limit to 2 servings a day	**High oxalates** (> 10 mg per serving) Avoid
Legumes, nuts, and seeds:		
Coconut	Cashews	Waxed green beans
Lentils	Garbanzo beans	Baked beans in
Water chestnuts	(1/4 cup cooked	tomato sauce
	Lima beans	Peanuts,
	Split peas	peanut butter
	Sunflower seeds	Pecans
	Walnuts	Tofu

Dr. Ina Wong, BSc, ND, RAc
#8 - 310 Goldstream Avenue
Victoria, B.C. Canada V9B 2W3

CHAPTER SEVEN

LOW OXALATE MENU IDEAS AND FOOD SWAPS

It takes some time to become familiar with the oxalate content of foods. The following menu ideas and food swaps will make it easier to adjust to a low oxalate diet. Some foods like spinach, beets, wheat and rice bran, almonds, and dark chocolate will have to be eliminated, but there are good substitutes for these foods. All other foods can safely be incorporated in the low oxalate diet. You will have to keep your daily oxalate consumption between 40-50 mg which means keeping track of the oxalate content of foods. When you consume medium or high oxalate foods pay careful attention to portion size. Most of your diet should be based on low or no oxalate foods.

Menu Ideas

Breakfasts

Eggs and Omelets (without high oxalate vegetables)

Pancakes (made with white rice flour or coconut flour)
Meats (avoid processed meats)
Yogurt with Fruit (choose low oxalate fruits)
Smoothies with Yogurt, Whey, or Banana (or any low oxalate fruit)
Avocado, Egg and Cream Cheese Omelet
Muffins (plain, banana, or pumpkin made with rice flour or coconut flour)

Lunch and Dinners

Basically any meat or fish with low oxalate vegetables and/or white rice
Salads (without spinach)
Stews or Soups (without high oxalate vegetables)
Spaghetti with White Rice Pasta
Tacos or Taco Salads
Pizza (made with low oxalate crust)
Chili (made with black eyed peas)

Snacks

Fruit (eliminating those on the high oxalate list)
Pumpkin Seeds
Avocado
Cheese (all varieties)
Corn Tortilla Chips with Cheese or Guacamole
Boiled or Deviled Eggs
Plain Bagel with Cream Cheese and/or Egg
Popcorn
Onion Rings (delicious fried in coconut oil)

Deserts

Breads, Cakes, and Cookies made with Coconut and/or Rice Flour
Banana Pudding

Vanilla Ice Cream
Yogurt
White Chocolate
Cheesecake

Food Swaps: High Oxalate - Low

Almond Milk – Cow Milk, Goat Milk or Coconut Milk
Beans – Black Eyed Peas
Spinach – Bok Choy and Romaine
Green Bell Peppers – Red or Yellow Bell Peppers
All Potatoes – Peeled Red Potatoes
Chocolate – White Chocolate
Brewed Tea – Instant Tea
Black Pepper – White Pepper
Whole Wheat Flour (plain or all purpose) – Regular, rice, coconut, or Tapioca Flour
Brown Rice – White Rice or Cauliflower Rice
Nuts and Seeds – Pumpkin Seeds
Spaghetti or Tomato Sauce – Alfredo Sauce
Whole Grain Pasta – Rice Pasta, Egg Noodles or Spiralized Zucchini
Potato Chips – Popcorn
Mashed Sweet Potatoes – Pumpkin or Butternut Squash
Peanut or Walnut Oil – Olive or Coconut Oil
Orange – Tangerine

Some quick and easy favorites at my house:

Cheddar or Parmesan Crisps
Sprinkle shredded cheese in a thin layer of rounds in a hot skillet and turn them when they've browned. These crispy thins can also be topped with avocado or sliced tomato.

Greek Salad

Finely chop 1 large cucumber, 1 Roma tomato, and crumble feta cheese. Add 1 tbsp. oregano, 1 tsp. white pepper, and 4 tbsp. extra virgin olive oil. Mix and serve, or serve as a dip with tortilla chips.

Cheesy Mashed Cauliflower

Olive Oil, Garlic, Chives, Romano Cheese, and mashed cauliflower.

Fried Artichokes

I can or frozen bag artichoke hearts drained and rinsed, coated with rice flour and fried in a small amount of olive oil.

Cherry Ice Cream

16 oz. frozen cherries and 1 ½ cup vanilla whole milk yogurt. Add to a food processor and process until smooth. The frozen cherries turn the yogurt to a soft serve ice cream. Can be frozen as well.

ABOUT THE AUTHOR

Melinda Keen is an author, middle school teacher and certified nutrition consultant. Her published works included *Mud in My Heart* (2007) a young adult novel, *Low Oxalate Fresh and Fast Cookbook* (2015) and *Real Food Real Results* (2016). *Low Oxalate Fresh and Fast Cookbook* contains a collection of meals that are perfect for the cook who wants home-cooked, nutritious, fresh food fast. Each recipe is low in oxalates to help heal symptoms of bladder pain, kidney stones, irritable bowel syndrome, fibromyalgia, and pain associated with oxalate stone formation in other parts of the body. It's a prevention diet often recommended for kidney stone issues. *Real Food Real Results: Gluten-Free, Low-Oxalate, Nutrient-Rich Recipes*, is an original collection of recipes from breakfasts to breads and crackers, main dishes and sides, and desserts.

BIBLIOGRAPHY

1. Lorenz EC, Michet CJ, Milliner DS, Lieske JC. (2013). Update on Oxalate Crystal Disease. Current rheumatology reports. 2013;15(7):340. doi:10.1007/s11926-013-0340-4.

2. Tristan Pascart, Pascal Richette, and René-Marc Flipo. (2014). Treatment of Nongout Joint Deposition Diseases: An Update Arthritis Volume 2014 Article ID 375202, 8 pages http://dx.doi.org/10.1155/2014/375202

3. Brasher WM, Zimmerman ER, Collings CK. (1969). The effects of prednisolone, indomethacin, and Aloe vera gel on tissue culture cells. Oral Surgery, Oral Medicine, Oral Pathology 1969, 27; 1: 122-128. https://www.sciencedirect.com/science/article/pii/0030422069900395

4. http://bioindividualnutrition.com/oxalates-their-influence-on-chronic-disease/

5. National Institutes of Health, U.S. Department of Health and Human Services. Opportunities and Challenges in Digestive Diseases Research: Recommendations of the National

Commission on Digestive Diseases. Bethesda, MD: National Institutes of Health; (2009). NIH Publication 08–6514

6. Mahboube Ganji-Arjenaki, Hamid Nasri, and Mahmoud Rafieian-Kopaei. (2017). Nephrolithiasis as a common urinary system manifestation of inflammatory bowel diseases; a clinical review and meta-analysis Journal of Nephrology. 2017 Apr 12. doi: 10.15171/jnp.2017.42

7. Tatta, Joe PT, DPT. (April 7, 2016). Ouch! Oxalates and Pain. http://www.drjoetatta.com/ouch-oxalates-and-pain/

8. Lorenz, E. C., Michet, C. J., Milliner, D. S., & Lieske, J. C. (2013). Update on Oxalate Crystal Disease. Current Rheumatology Reports, 15(7), 340. http://doi.org/10.1007/s11926-013-0340-4

9. Brock,Deborah A. Hundley, Janice M. (1995). Identifying Calcium Oxalate Crystals in Urine, Laboratory Medicine, Volume 26, Issue 11, 1 November 1995, Pages 733–735. https://doi.org/10.1093/labmed/26.11.733

10. Haefner, Hope K., MD. Management of the Patient with Vulvar Pain Syndromes Study Resource Handout. www.studyres.com

11 Lorenz, E. C., Michet, C. J., Milliner, D. S., & Lieske, J. C. (2013). Update on Oxalate Crystal Disease. Current Rheumatology Reports, 15(7), 340. http://doi.org/10.1007/s11926-013-0340-4)

12. Lorenz, E. C., Michet, C. J., Milliner, D. S., & Lieske, J. C. (2013). Update on Oxalate Crystal Disease. Current Rheumatology Reports, 15(7), 340. http://doi.org/10.1007/s11926-013-0340-4

13. Oxalosis Children's Hospital St. Louis. http://www.stlouischildrens.org/diseases-conditions/oxalosis

14. Morrison, Clare. (August 14, 2014). Ditch Healthy Berries to Beat Muscle Pain: The Eating Plan That Helped Me Cure My Aches and Pains. http://www.dailymail.co.uk/health/article-2187890

15. Help Prevent Kidney Stones with a Low-Oxalate Diet UROLOGY. (January 13, 2016). University of Pittsburgh Medical Center. http://share.upmc.com/2016/01/help-prevent-kidney-stones-with-a-low-oxalate-diet/

16. Weiwen Chai and Michael Liebman. (2005). Effect of Different Cooking Methods on Vegetable Oxalate Content Journal of Agricultural and Food Chemistry. March 18, 2005 DOI: 10.1021/jf048128d. http://pubs.acs.org/doi/abs/10.1021/jf048128

17. Bankhead, Charles. (2013). Light Exercise Still Cuts Kidney Stone Risk. https://www.medpagetoday.com May 05, 2013.

18. Sanchari Sinha, Som Nath Singh, Y.P. Monga, and Uday Sankar Ray. (2007). Improvement of Glutathione and Total Antioxidant Status with Yoga The Journal of Alternative and Complementary Medicine. December 2007, Vol. 13, No. 10: 1085-1090. http://online.liebertpub.com/doi/pdf/10.1089/acm.2007.0567)

19. National Kidney Foundation. (2016). A-Z Health Guide Calcium Oxalate Stones. May 16.

20. The Environmental Working Group (EWG). (2017). The 2017 Dirty Dozen: Strawberries, spinach Top EWG's List of Pesticides in Produce. March 8.

21. The Environmental Working Group (EWG). (July 15, 2014). Is Organic Really Better?

22. United States Department of Agriculture Recent Trends in GE Adoption. https://www.ers.usda.gov/data-products/adoption-of-genetically-engineered-crops-in-the-us/recent-trends-in-ge-adoption.aspx

23. Penniston, KL, Steele, TH, Nakada, SY. (2007). Lemonade therapy increases urinary citrate and urine volumes in patients with recurrent calcium oxalate stone formation. US National Library of Medicine National Institutes of Health Urology. Nov;70(5):856-60. Epub 2007 Oct 24. https://www.ncbi.nlm.nih.gov/pubmed/17919696/)

24. Arthritis Foundation, Best Fish For Arthritis. http://www.arthritis.org/living-with-arthritis/arthritis-diet/best-foods-for-arthritis/best-fish-for-arthritis.php

25. Siener, R, et al. Effect of n-3 fatty acid supplementation on urinary risk factors for calcium oxalate stone formation. (2011). Journal of Urology, Vol. 185, February 2011, pp. 719-24.

26. Cuesta, Stephanie. (April 1, 2017). Health Tips Osteroporosis, Cholesterol..! Sound Familiar? Vitamin K2 Should Too. http://www.stephcuesta.com

27. Baxmann, AC, De O G Mendonça C, HeilberKidney Int. (2003). Mar;63(3):1066-71. Effect of vitamin C supplements on urinary oxalate and pH in calcium stone-forming patients. IP Kidney Int. 2003 Mar;63(3):1066-71. https://www.ncbi.nlm.nih.gov/pubmed/12631089

28. Science Daily, American Society of Nephrology. (2013). Calcium Supplementation May Increase The Risk of Kidney

Stone Recurrence October 13, 2015. https://www.sciencedaily.com/releases/2015/10/151013103619.htm

29. Schwille PO, Schmiedl A, Herrmann U, Fan J, Gottlieb D, Manoharan M, Wipplinger J. (1999). Magnesium, citrate, magnesium citrate and magnesium-alkali citrate as modulators of calcium oxalate crystallization in urine: observations in patients with recurrent idiopathic calcium urolithiasis. University Hospital Department of Surgery, Erlangen, Germany. Urol Res. 1999 Apr;27(2):117-26. https://www.ncbi.nlm.nih.gov/pubmed/10424393

30. Conlon, M. A., & Bird, A. R. (2015). The Impact of Diet and Lifestyle on Gut Microbiota and Human Health. Nutrients, 7(1), 17–44. http://doi.org/10.3390/nu7010017

31. Waring R.H., Klovrza L.V. (2000). Sulphur Metabolism in Autism. Journal of Nutritional and Environmental Medicine 10, 25–32.

32. Eck P, Friel J. (2013). Should Probiotics be considered as Vitamin Supplements? Vitam Miner 3: e124. doi:10.4172/vms.1000e124.

33. Duncan, S. H., Richardson, A. J., Kaul, P., Holmes, R. P., Allison, M. J., & Stewart, C. S. (2002). Oxalobacter formigenes and Its Potential Role in Human Health. Applied and Environmental Microbiology, 68(8), 3841–3847. http://doi.org/10.1128/AEM.68.8.3841-3847.2002

34 Scott, Karen. (2017). ANTIBIOTICS: USE WITH International Scientific Association For Probiotics And Prebiotics. FEBRUARY 24, 2017. https://isappscience.org/antibiotics-use-caution/

35. Duncan, S. H., Richardson, A. J., Kaul, P., Holmes, R. P., Allison, M. J., & Stewart, C. S. (2002). Oxalobacter formigenes and Its Potential Role in Human Health. Applied and Environmental Microbiology, 68(8), 3841–3847. http://doi.org/10.1128/AEM.68.8.3841-3847.2002

36 Gantz, Matthew. CEO of OxThera AB.http://www.oxathera.com

37. http://nutritiondata.self.com/facts/recipe/2422683/2

38. Knight, J. Jiang J,Assimos, D.G., Holmes, R.P. (2006). Hydroxyproline ingestion and urinary oxalate and glycolate excretion. Kidney International Official Journal of the International Society of Nephrology. published online 4 October 2006. http://www.kidney-international.theisn.org/article/S0085-2538(15)51883-8/fulltext)

39. Pragasam V, Kalaiselvi P, Sumitra K, Srinivasan S, Varalakshmi P. (2005). Counteraction of oxalate induced nitrosative stress by supplementation of l-arginine, a potent antilithic agent. The National Center for Biotechnology Information Apr;354(1-2):159-66. Epub 2005 Jan 19. http://pubmed/15748613

40. Byer K, Khan SR. (2005). Citrate provides protection against oxalate and calcium oxalate crystal induced oxidative damage to renal epithelium. The National Center for Biotechnology Feb;173(2):640-6. https://www.ncbi.nlm.nih.gov/pubmed/15643280

41. Penniston, Kristina. UW Hospital Metabolic Stone Clinic Citric Acid and Kidney Stones.

42. Harvard T.H. Chan School of Public Health Nutrition Data compiled with the assistance of UAB - School of Medicine - Urology - Ross Holmes, Ph.D. https://regepi.bwh.harvard.edu/health/Oxalate/files

43. Wichita Nephrology Group Patient Education. https://wichitanephrology.com

44. University of Pittsburg Medical Center. UROLOGY. (2016). Health and Wellness Help Prevent Kidney Stones with a Low-Oxalate Diet, January 13, 2016. http://www.upmc.com/pages/default.aspx

45. Wong, Ina. NATUROPATHIC PHYSICIAN REGISTERED ACUPUNCTURIST. Patient Handouts Oxalate Content of Foods. http://www.drwong.ca/

Made in the USA
Las Vegas, NV
02 November 2023